REAL FOOD FERMENTATION

for Beginners

Quarto.com

First Published in 2025 by New Shoe Press, an imprint of The Quarto Group,
100 Cummings Center, Suite 265-D, Beverly, MA 01915, USA.
T (978) 282-9590 F (978) 283-2742

Essential, In-Demand Topics, Four-Color Design, Affordable Price
New Shoe Press publishes affordable, beautifully designed books covering evergreen, in-demand subjects. With a goal to inform and inspire readers' everyday hobbies, from cooking and gardening to wellness and health to art and crafts, New Shoe titles offer the ultimate library of purposeful, how-to guidance aimed at meeting the unique needs of each reader. Reimagined and redesigned from Quarto's best-selling backlist, New Shoe books provide practical knowledge and opportunities for all DIY enthusiasts to enrich and enjoy their lives.

Visit Quarto.com/New-Shoe-Press for a complete listing of the New Shoe Press books.

New Shoe Press titles are also available at discount for retail, wholesale, promotional, and bulk purchase. For details, contact the Special Sales Manager by email at specialsales@quarto.com or by mail at The Quarto Group, Attn: Special Sales Manager, 100 Cummings Center, Suite 265-D, Beverly, MA 01915, USA.

10 9 8 7 6 5 4 3 2 1

ISBN: 978-0-7603-9802-9
eISBN: 978-0-7603-9803-6

The content in this book was previously published in *Real Food Fermentation, Revised and Expanded* (Quarry Books 2022) by Alex Lewin.

Library of Congress Cataloging-in-Publication Data available

Page Layout: *tabula rasa* graphic design
Photography: Glenn Scott Photography, except Nader Khouri pages 64–67, 122–137; Shutterstock page 115

Printed in China

The information in this book is for educational purposes only. It is not intended to replace the advice of a physician or medical practitioner. Please see your health-care provider before beginning any new health program.

REAL FOOD FERMENTATION
for Beginners

Preserving Whole Fresh Food with Live Cultures in Your Home Kitchen

ALEX LEWIN

NEW SHOE PRESS

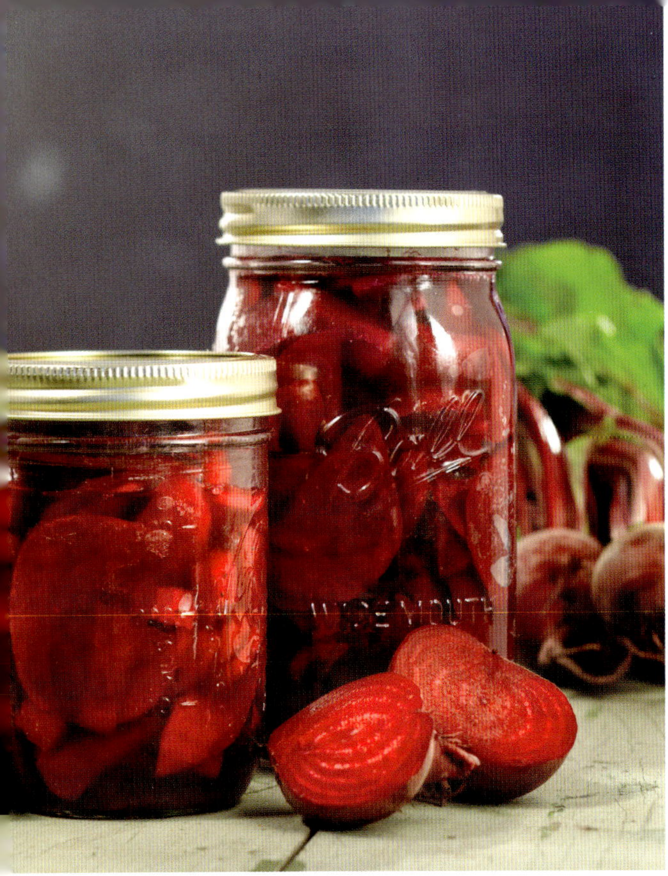
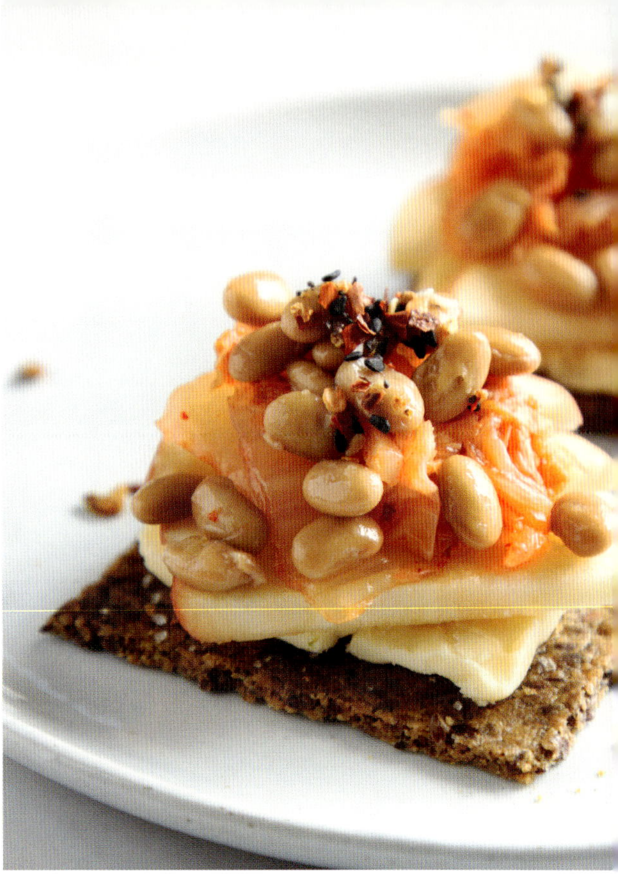
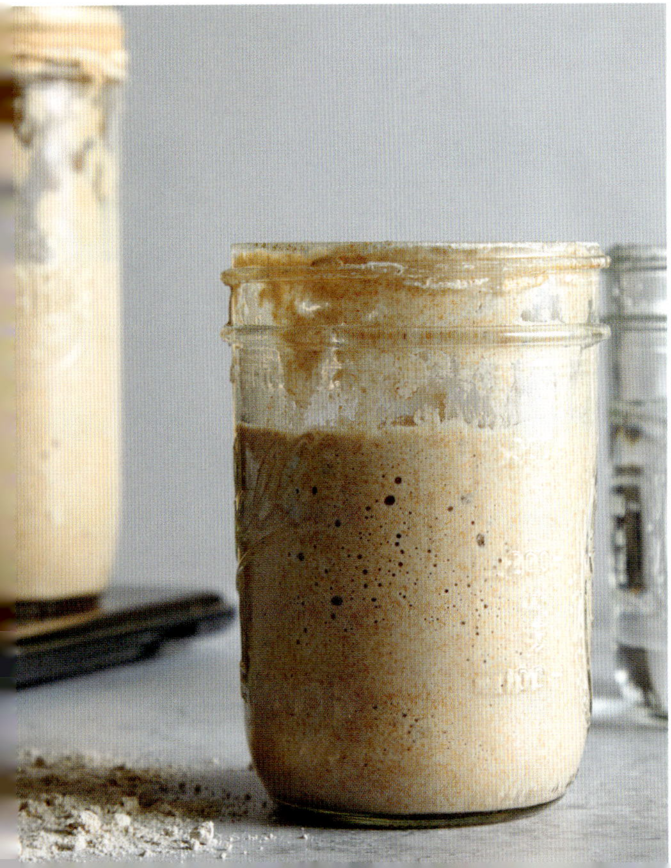
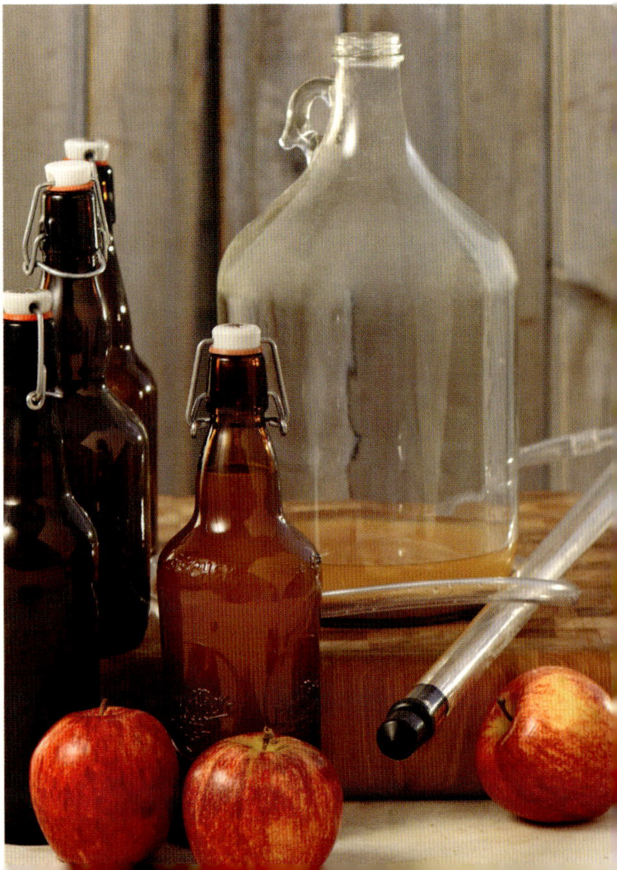

Contents

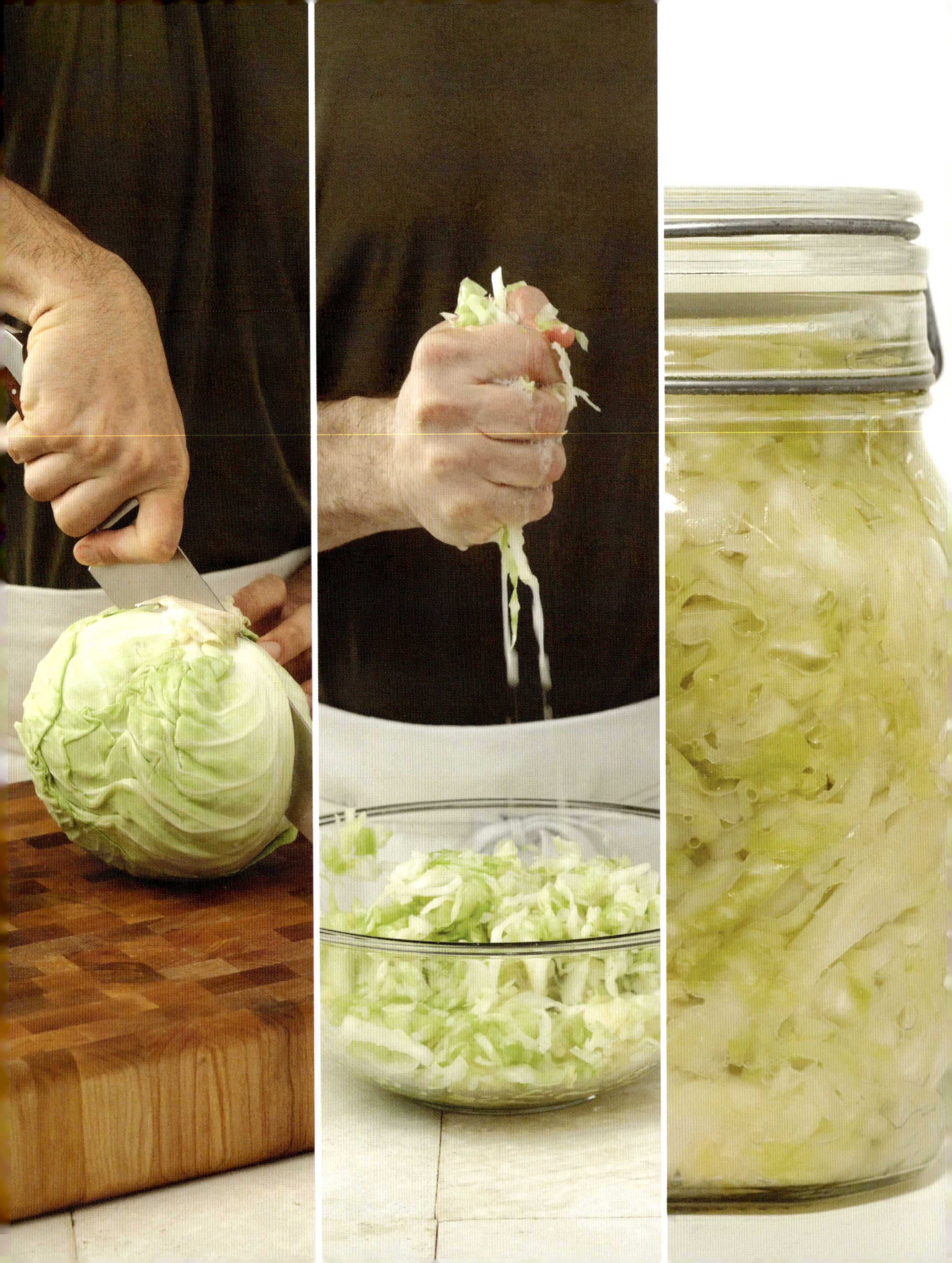

INTRODUCTION

Fermentation Journey

I like changing things for the better. I am curious about how things work. And I think a lot about food.

I love the idea of transforming food, in harmony with nature, as it has been done for thousands of years. Sauerkraut, for instance, need contain nothing more than cabbage and salt—no mysterious chemicals, no additives, not even any vinegar. So simple, yet so complex: Fermentation occurs because we seduce microscopic beings into doing our biochemical bidding, and they create sour acids that can preserve cabbage for many seasons.

I also love the process of making fermented foods. It is a checklist of gratifying activities. I go to a farmers' market or a farm, chat with food producers, and pay them a fair price for their work. I think creatively about what food I want to make. I craft the food myself, using whatever tools are available, sometimes improvising, and I often wind up with something great. In time, I get the reward of eating it and of sharing it with my community of friends and family.

When we make our own food, we regain some control over our lives, which is especially important at a time in history when many of us feel at the mercy of events, governments, corporations, and industrial food producers. We also bridge the global gulf between the people who make food and the people who eat it, a gulf that perpetuates a grim litany of problems from famine and obesity to pollution, water shortages, wars over scarce resources, and deforestation.

I am delighted to share with you my passion for fermentation.

Take what you want from this book, experiment, and set out on your own food journey so that you might transform your food, your world, and yourself.

How to Use This Book

Each chapter has a specific focus. The first chapter is an overview of food preserving. Chapter 2 discusses choosing ingredients. Chapter 3 provides an in-depth look at making sauerkraut and broadens to other fermented vegetables. The remaining chapters walk you through fermenting dairy, fruit condiments, beverages, and sourdough.

Perhaps all you want to do is make fermented fruit chutney. With a typical cookbook, you might simply turn to the chutney recipe and follow it without reading the rest of the chapter. With this book, I encourage you to skim the whole chapter, or even the whole book, first! Knowledge is cumulative, and points made earlier in the book inform the recipes throughout.

People read books, especially cookbooks, in their own way. And many people don't want to be told how to read a book. But I do have reasons for making my suggestions.

If I've done my job right, then the early chapters will give you information to help you understand why the recipes work, some peace of mind about why they are safe, a better idea of what to do when things go wrong, and tools to help you decide how you might or might not want to modify the recipes as you continue to make them.

Recipes in some chapters depend on ingredients that you make in other chapters. When this is the case, I point it out, so of course you can jump back and forth and read the relevant sections as needed. Fermented fruit condiments, for instance, require a starter, and making sauerkraut and straining yogurt are two good ways to get a starter. If you've already read about making sauerkraut and straining yogurt, you will understand the starters you need for making fruit condiments. If you haven't, you might need to go back and read those sections again.

The more you have thought about the sources of your ingredients, the more satisfaction you may get out of a recipe, and in some cases, the better the recipe will work—and the healthier it will be. For this reason, you may find it useful to read the chapter about selecting ingredients, chapter 2, before you try any of the recipes. For instance, it is good to understand when chlorinated water can be a problem, along with ways that you can remove chlorine from water; when it's most important to avoid pesticide-treated fruit; and the relative merits of different kinds of salt.

Preserving Food

Preserving food is an important aspect of food preparation. Food can be preserved in many ways. Some preserving methods are suitable for home, while others are feasible only in an industrial setting.

- Drying and salting are two of the oldest preserving methods. All the method-specific ingredients are easy to get: salt, heat, and fresh air. Many types of food can be dried and/or salted, including fruits, grains, and fish and meats. In fact, humans have been growing grain for at least 10,000 years, and because growing grain does not make sense unless you dry it, we can conclude that humans have been drying food for at least 10,000 years.
- Ultraviolet light, ionizing radiation, and high pressure are some of the newest tools for preserving food. Some food you buy in the store has been processed with these technologies: nuts and spices are often irradiated, for instance, and prepared foods like guacamole are sometimes treated with high pressure. These are not preserving techniques that you can employ at home.

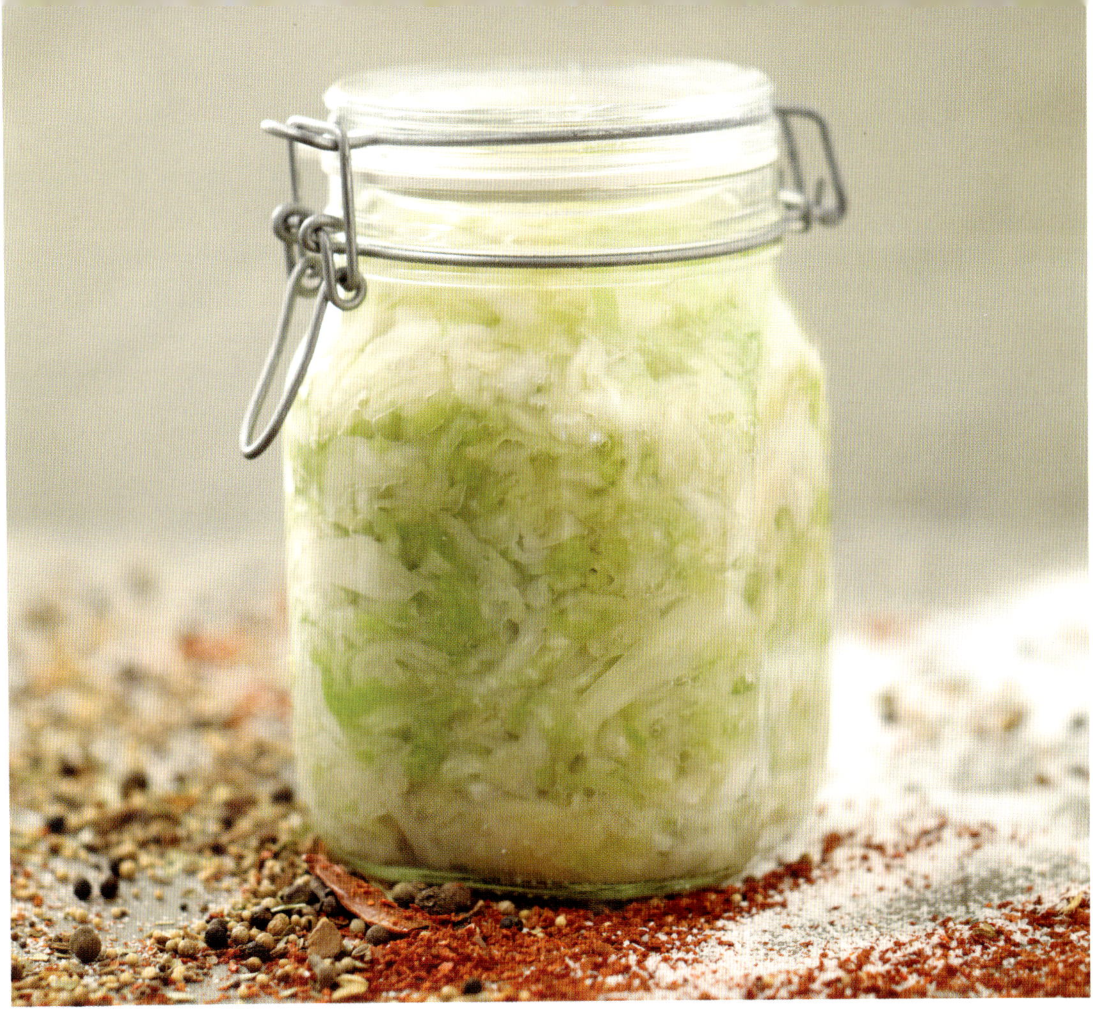

- Vinegar, acids like citric acid or ascorbic acid, and other preservative chemicals can be added to foods to help them remain edible longer. Home preservers use these additives, as do industrial food producers. Some preservative chemicals, such as sodium nitrite, may be harmful to our health.
- Canning is a food preserving technique that was invented in the early 1800s. It is a popular and practical way to preserve food, on both a small and a large scale. It is often used in conjunction with vinegar, acids, and other preservative chemicals.
- Refrigeration is another popular food preserving technique. Before electricity was widely available, ice suppliers cut big blocks of ice from frozen lakes and shipped them to warmer areas, where they would be used to keep food cold. Things are easier today, at least in wealthy countries with electricity.
- Freezing is one of the most popular long-term food preserving techniques today. It often requires a steady supply of electricity. It's only in the last hundred years that freezing food at home has become practical year-round. Many people freeze food every day without thinking of it as a preserving technique.

Fermenting: My Favorite Food Preserving Technique

Fermenting, last and definitely not least, is my favorite food preserving method. It is peculiarly well suited to the home food preserver and has been for a long time, in rich countries and in poor ones. Here's why:

Fermenting is tolerant of imprecision. Fermentation can succeed even when there's variation in times, temperatures, and ingredient ratios. It is pretty difficult to get food poisoning from wrongly fermented foods.

Canning, by contrast, is much less tolerant of im-precision; it is a persnickety process, and failure to sterilize equipment properly, or to process canned food for the right length of time or at the right temperatures, can lead to serious food poisoning often with no telltale signs. This food poisoning is relatively rare these days because proper procedures are well documented and understood, but the specter of food poisoning makes me less inclined to improvise when canning—and that takes some of the fun out of it for me.

Fermentation generally does not require expensive or unusual equipment, often requiring no special equipment whatsoever. Many vegetable fermentation recipes rely only on vegetables, salt, a knife, and jars. Some recipes can be facilitated or expedited by the use of a food processor—making kimchi with only a knife, or with a mortar and pestle, can be time consuming, for instance—but power tools are never necessary. Fermentation can always be achieved without electricity, often without any source of energy at all besides arms and hands (and sometimes feet). Some fermentation recipes require a degree of temperature control, but the requirement is generally approximate and can be achieved via low-tech means.

Fermentation can be self-perpetuating. When fermentation recipes do require special ingredients, they are often ingredients that can be created via fermentation. Because of this, fermentation is more sustainable, in the literal sense, than processes that require ingredients that might be hard to find, now or in the future, or that require industrial manufacturing. Many people made cider and wine before it was possible to buy packets of yeast in the store. Packets of yeast can save you time or trouble, but they are not necessary and can sometimes diminish the sense of adventure.

Fermentation can enhance the nutritive value, healthfulness, and digestibility of foods. The microbes responsible for fermentation often create enzymes and vitamins, break down difficult-to-digest food components, and make minerals more bioavailable. Fermentation is the best preserving method in this regard.

Beyond all of this, fermentation involves an element of magic, and an element of faith. In order to ferment our food, we conjure armies of invisible microbes to wage war against the forces of decay. We create the right conditions for them, by arranging for the right amount of salt, the right amount of air, the right temperature, and so on, and we must trust that the soldiers will arrive and ferment. Even in today's world of high-speed Internet and GPS navigation, I still get a little thrill each time my sauerkraut starts bubbling because I know that it means I have successfully seduced the microbes.

ARCHETYPES OF FERMENTATION

CATEGORY	MICROBES	ARCHETYPE	OTHER EXAMPLES
Lacto-fermented vegetables, fruit, berries, and buds	Bacteria	Sauerkraut	Cucumber pickles, kimchi, fermented vegetables, preserved lemons, olives, capers and caperberries, salsas, chutneys
Lacto-fermented vegetable brines	Bacteria	Beet kvass	Root beer, vegetable kvass, and other beverages fermented with whey and fermented vegetable juice as starters
Fermented dairy	Bacteria (mostly), yeast, mold	Yogurt	Kefir, crème fraîche, sour cream, cultured butter, aged cheese
Alcoholic beverages	Yeast (mostly)	Hard apple cider	Wine, beer, mead
Dual-fermented beverages	Bacteria, yeast	Vinegar	Kombucha, dairy kefir, water kefir
"Exotic" foods	Bacteria (mostly)	Chocolate	Coffee, vanilla, aged tea
Fermented soy	Various	Soy sauce	Miso, tempeh, natto
Fermented grains and starches	Bacteria, yeast	Bread	Sour porridges, poi, fufu, injera

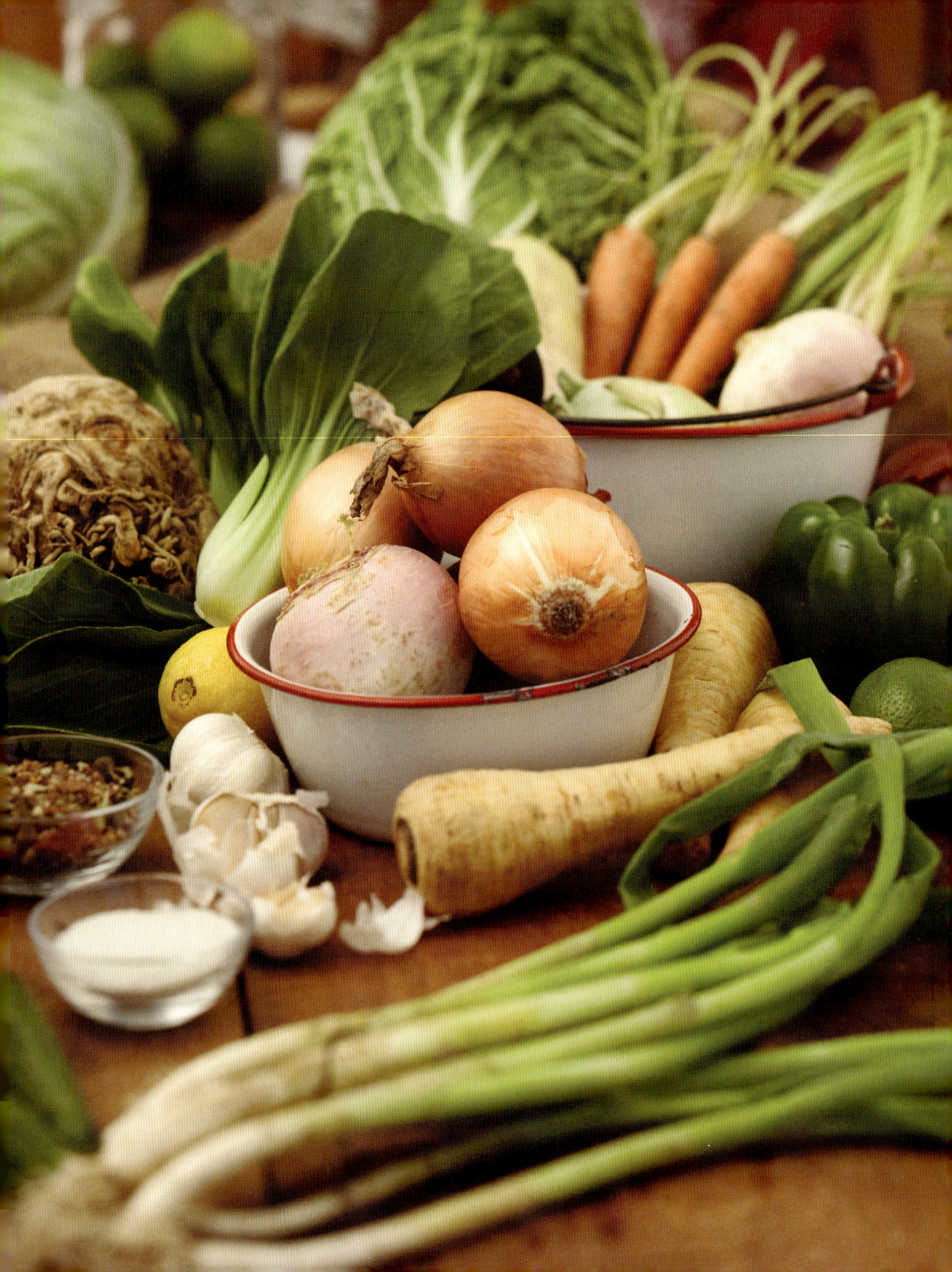

CHAPTER 1

Food Preserving (In Brief)

This chapter discusses what it means for food to spoil—both how we experience spoiled food and what processes cause it to spoil. Food preserving is everything that we do to prevent food from spoiling or to slow down the process. The conditions that cause food to spoil can be analyzed and broken down into various factors; I'll discuss each of these, as well as how you might seek to adjust them to postpone spoilage. Understanding all of these things will help you understand the mechanisms whereby various popular food preserving techniques, particularly fermentation, work.

It is worthwhile to look at food preserving in a somewhat technical and quantitative way; this helps us see why our preserved food is safe and how we can modify our recipes without compromising safety. For instance, if we know that acidity preserves food, we may feel comfortable replacing vinegar with lemon juice or kombucha in a recipe.

What Is Food Preserving?

Food preserving is *extending a food's window of edibility*. Edibility has to do with safety and palatability (including deliciousness).

Left to its own devices, food tends to spoil, more or less quickly depending on its type. A head of cabbage left out on the kitchen counter, for instance, might go some number of days before starting to dry out; insects might start to eat it, and, depending on the temperature and humidity, it might start to get moldy. In the summer, it certainly wouldn't be very appetizing after maybe five days. By comparison, fermented cabbage can last weeks, months, or years at room temperature. Sailors used to take sauerkraut on long ocean voyages, and in Korea, kimchi is made in the fall and then eaten all winter and spring.

Fruit is still more perishable than cabbage: raspberries, for instance, can get moldy in less than a day, and peaches shrivel up even while getting mushy. Fresh grapes are best right after they've been picked and are pretty unappealing after sitting out for a couple of weeks, but wine can have a shelf life of anywhere from one year to fifty years!

When trying to extend a food's window of edibility, you face challenges from a few sources:

Other organisms that try to eat your food. Organisms, large and small, mammalian, single-celled, and everything in between, will try to eat your food. These organisms can range from rodents and insects to yeasts, molds, and bacteria. Depending on where you are, you may even be in competition with deer, coyotes, eagles, or bears. Some of these organisms are more visible than others. In fact, the microscopic ones live everywhere—in the air and the water and even on your skin. Preventing them from eating your food can be difficult. Often the best you can hope for is to choose which ones will win.

Ancient Means, Modern Reasons

While food preserving originated as a survival technique, and later became essential for travel and commerce, people gradually discovered and rediscovered that preserved food can be different from the original, and sometimes better.

New textures and flavors develop; wine, cheese, and bread are excellent examples. Digestive and nutritive benefits accrue; many preserved foods, such as fermented cassava (versus raw cassava), sauerkraut (versus raw cabbage), and natto (versus raw soybeans), are easier to digest and more nutritious than their fresh counterparts, sometimes dramatically so. In fact, raw soybeans and raw cassava can be toxic!

Cellular breakdown. In a living plant or animal, as quickly as old cells die off, break down, and are reabsorbed, new cells are created. The breakdown is catalyzed by enzymes, and the creation of new cells is made possible by the circulation throughout the body of energy and cellular building blocks. When an animal dies or a vegetable or fruit is picked, this circulation stops, so the existing cells continue to break down, but no new cells are created to replace them. The cellular breakdown manifests itself as the loss of water from cells and the weakening of cell walls. This is part of why old vegetables dry out or become mushy. Greens lose their crunchiness, tomatoes and other soft fruit get softer, and summer squash start to cave in.

Oxidation. Some foods are subject to oxidation when exposed to air. We see this when we cut a piece of raw meat or an avocado, an apple, or a potato, and it starts turning brown.

WHY PRESERVE?

Why would we want to extend a food's window of edibility? There are many reasons why, historically, we have preserved food, and will continue to preserve it:

- Hunter-gatherers of the past (as nearly all of them are) devoted relatively little time to food preserving; for the most part, they ate what was available, when it was available. If they could not find enough to eat in a given place, they moved somewhere else, or sometimes they suffered. If we preserve food, then we don't have to move when we run out of local, seasonal food.
- The advent of agriculture, grains in particular, drew into sharp focus the problem of the uneven yield cycle: Much of the crop would be ready for harvest all at once, and there would be long gaps between harvests. This was particularly the case for people living in colder climates, where entire seasons go by with no new crops. Raising livestock for meat brought similar issues: It is better to have weeks or months to eat a cow, rather than being forced to eat it all at once. Thus, preserving allows food from a bounty to be consumed gradually.
- When people started keeping animals for milk, the need arose for a way to preserve dairy products, since milk does not remain fresh very long in warm weather. This need led to the emergence of a broad range of dairy foods, including yogurt, kefir, butter, cheese, and so on. Most dairy foods can be looked at as "preserved milk" because they have a much longer room-temperature life expectancy than milk.
- Explorers, travelers, and specifically sailors have always had to carry supplies to last for weeks or months. At some point, people figured out that they needed a variety of foods in order to avoid diseases of deficiency; for instance, sailors started bringing with them citrus juice, sauerkraut, and other foods containing vitamin C because vitamin C is protective against scurvy. Today's astronauts, whose diets are limited to what they take with them on their ships, have the same needs. Food preserving has allowed humans to travel places they could not otherwise have reached.
- As explorers traveled the world and societies mingled, demand arose for goods from faraway places, "exotic" goods that needed to be transported thousands of miles. (The word "exotic" derives from the Greek *exotikos*, meaning simply "from outside.") Tea and sugar cane are good examples; their monetary value and great popularity created a compelling incentive for their preservation and transportation.
- Even small amounts of alcohol are quite effective at killing potentially harmful microorganisms—and alcoholic beverages are products of fermentation. Thus, when safe drinking water has been scarce, as it has been in many places since the advent of sedentary agriculture and the dawn of cities, mild alcoholic beverages have been a useful option.

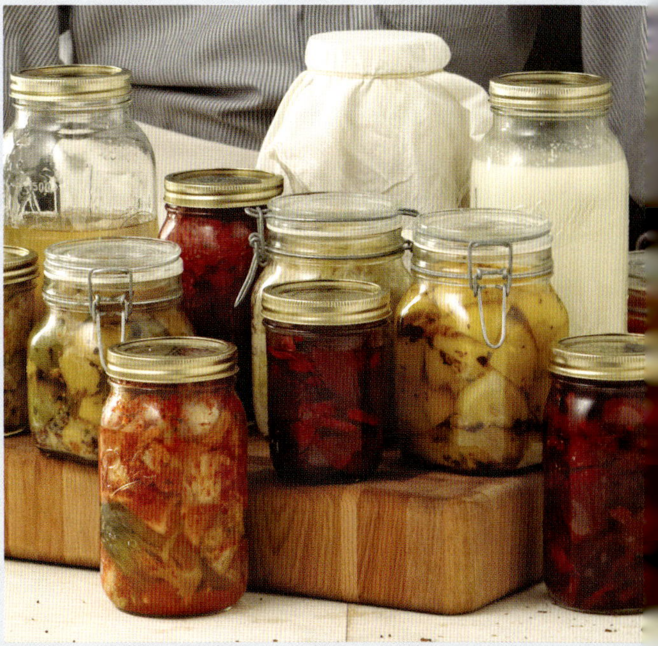

SOME SIGNATURE FERMENTED FOODS

(*Note:* The regions listed are not necessarily the regions of origin.)

REGION/CULTURE	TRADEMARK FOOD	INGREDIENTS
Central and Eastern Europe and East Asia	Sauerkraut	Cabbage, salt, and spices
Asia and Eastern Europe	Yogurt and kefir	Milk
Korea	Kimchi	Cabbage, salt, and spices
Europe and Mediterranean and Asia	Ham and dry sausage	Pork and salt
Europe and West Asia	Wine	Grapes
Europe, Africa	Beer	Grain
Northern Europe and North America	Cider	Apples
Europe and Mediterranean	Cheese	Milk and rennet
Japan	Miso	Soybeans
East Asia	Soy Sauce	Soybeans
Mediterranean, Southeast Asia	Preserved citrus	Citrus and salt
Southeast Asia, East Asia	Fish sauce	Fish and salt
Many places	Bread	Wheat and water
Ethiopia and other equatorial and subtropical regions	Coffee	

Ways to Delay Decay

Different preserving methods use different strategies to fend off decay. These are some of the methods that can be used by the home preserver:

- Refrigeration and freezing are effective because most microbes' metabolisms, and the actions of enzymes, slow greatly in the cold and essentially stop below freezing. Refrigeration and freezing do not gravely compromise the nutritional content of food, although the freeze/thaw cycle can burst food cell walls, affecting texture.
- Packing in an acidic environment is a quick, cheap, and effective way of preserving food. This can be done via fermentation or by adding vinegar. Most microbes and enzymes cannot operate in a highly acidic environment. Other chemical preservatives such as sodium benzoate are sometimes used alongside acids. Some of these preservative chemicals may be harmful to us.
- Packing in alcohol is another way to preserve food. A high-alcohol environment is effectively a low-moisture environment; microbes and enzymes are disabled or destroyed.
- Drying, salting, and sugaring are ways of drawing water out of food, rendering it insufficiently wet for the activities of many kinds of microbes and enzymes.
- Canning, whether in metal cans or in glass jars, relies on heat to destroy all microbes and enzymes, and relies on a hermetic seal to prevent microbes from reentering. The great virtue of canning is that when it is done properly, it can keep food for years. Its shortcomings are that (1) it can occasionally fail, and its failure can be disastrous, even fatal, because of the *Clostridium botulinum* (botulism) bacteria, and (2) the heat used in canning diminishes some heat-sensitive vitamins and destroys enzymes.
- Meat that has been cooked to remove much of its moisture, salted to remove more, and then immersed in fat to create an anaerobic environment is called confit. It can keep for months.
- Dairy has its own family of preservation techniques that variously convert sugars into acids, draw out water, isolate fat, and in some cases use heat to control bacteria and enzymes.
- Fermentation underlies many of the techniques already listed. Vinegar and alcohol are both products of fermentation, and most ways of preserving dairy involve fermentation.

NEW FRONTIERS IN FOOD PRESERVATION

New technologies, such as ultraviolet irradiation, high-pressure processing, and pulsed electric field processing, are now being used to sterilize food. Some of these technologies have been unleashed on the public after minimal testing and with little fanfare. Ideally, we could wait twenty years or so, see what unforeseen consequences emerge, weigh the costs and benefits, and then decide for ourselves which of these methods seem safe. Unfortunately, full disclosure is the exception rather than the rule, and unless we are acquiring food directly from its producer, it can be hard to tell how it may have been processed.

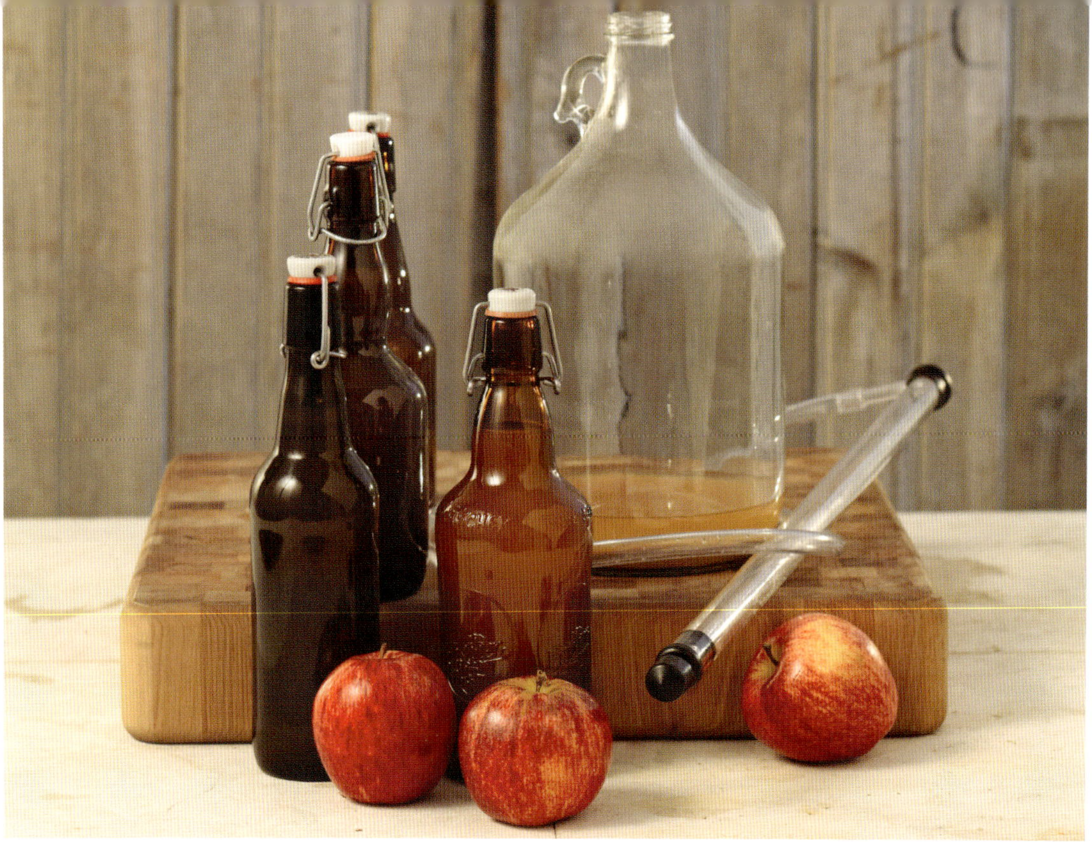

Cider-making equipment

Case Study: Apples

What are the possible fates of an apple?

If you let an apple drop from its tree, it will likely get eaten by worms, birds, small land animals, or large land animals (like bears!). Or, especially if it is damaged in its fall from the tree branch, it might succumb to bacteria, yeasts, and molds. The exposed flesh is also likely to oxidize (turn brown), and, depending on the weather conditions, the apple might start to shrivel and dry up.

If you like, you can create a brighter future for this apple.

First, you can pick it carefully and store it somewhere moist and cool or cold (but not freezing). Under the right conditions, fresh apples can be stored for months.

Alternatively, you can core and slice the apple, and then put it in a hot, dry place until it is dehydrated. You can dry it until its texture is like that of leather, or until it is like that of a potato chip, or somewhere in between. If you do this and keep it somewhere dry, it can last for months.

You can purée the apple, perhaps add some lemon juice, heat it, put it in a jar, heat it some more, and then put it on a shelf. By doing this, you will have canned it. It will keep for a very long time, but you will have lost more of its natural vitamins and enzymes than in any of these other scenarios.

Finally, you can ferment the apple. Depending on what you're interested in doing, you might mix the apple with other fruit or vegetables and spices, introduce the right kinds of bacteria, and thus produce a chutney. Or you might juice the apple, introduce some yeast (or cross your fingers), wait a week or two, and produce some nice hard apple cider.

Case Study: Cabbage

Consider the many different possible fates of a picked cabbage. The first, and least appetizing, option is to pick it and leave it out in the field on a warm day. There it may be partly eaten by animals or insects. It may also start to decompose, or rot, which is to say it may be partly eaten by microbes of various sorts or dissolved by its own enzymes.

As a home cook, you have these other options for processing the cabbage:

It can be cooled: If it is kept somewhere isolated at a low temperature, like in a refrigerator or a cellar, its rate of decay will be slowed greatly.

It can be canned: If it is heated and sealed under pressure in a sterile airtight container, it will reach a stable state that it might maintain for months or years.

It can be fermented: But if it is packed in salty liquid, and if other conditions are right, then it will follow a course that is a sort of middle road between rotting and canning—perhaps the best of both worlds. It will be eminently edible, and at the same time it will be a fertile playground for benign microbes. We call this fermentation.

Case Study: Milk

Most of us have been told not to leave milk out on the counter because it will spoil. This is a bit of an oversimplification of what happens, but regardless, there are other things you can do with milk besides keeping it out on the counter or putting it in the refrigerator.

If you skim the cream off the top of whole milk (assuming the milk has not been homogenized) and use just the cream, you can make butter, which will keep longer than milk.

If you introduce particular colonies of bacteria and then keep everything warm, you can make a durable, digestible, probiotic-rich, sour dairy food called yogurt.

By adding other things, heating it, separating the milk in various ways, and perhaps aging the result, you can produce a wide variety of other fermented dairy products, including cheeses.

BACTERIA VERSUS YEAST VERSUS BOTH

The term "microbe" can refer to any microscopic organism. The microbes responsible for many of our favorite fermented foods are bacteria and yeast. Some fermented foods (sake, some cheeses, some meat products, and some soy products) also rely on specific molds and other fungi to achieve their unique end points. Note that yeasts and molds are both types of fungi, along with mushrooms.

In general, yeasts consume sugars and produce alcohol, while bacteria consume sugars, starches, or alcohol and produce acids. Both alcohol and acids play roles in food preserving.

As foods become acidic, they become inhospitable to most kinds of microbes. Fortunately for us, the microbes that can survive in acidic environments are safe for us to eat: many of them are microbes that live within our bodies, and many of them are bacteria that enhance our digestion.

Food that contains more alcohol contains less water, which can make it less hospitable for some kinds of microbes. Also, alcohol itself is toxic to some microbes. In high enough concentrations, alcohol is toxic even to alcohol-producing yeasts, so 20 percent, or thereabouts, is the upper limit on alcohol content for a fermented beverage. To get a higher alcohol content than that, it's necessary to use the process of distillation, which separates the alcohol from the water by taking advantage of alcohol's lower boiling point. This is how stronger alcoholic beverages like brandy and vodka are made.

FAVORITE FERMENTED FOODS AND THEIR FAVORITE MICROBES

BACTERIA	YEAST	MOLD
Sauerkraut	Sake	Sake
Kimchi	Wine	Cheese (some)
Pickles	Beer	Soy sauce
Yogurt	Mead	Miso
Cheese (most)	Bread	Dry sausage
Kefir	Kefir	
Vinegar	Vinegar	
Kombucha	Kombucha	

An Overview of Fermentation: Getting to Know the Process

How exactly do you ferment food?

- First, you need the food medium itself, which usually contains some carbohydrates. This food may be vegetables or vegetable juice, fruits or fruit juice, grains, dairy, or even meat or fish. You can also add carbohydrates to foods (often in the form of sugar), and then ferment the result; kombucha, for instance, is made from sugar-sweetened tea.
- Next, you need the microbes, which you may get from any number of sources:
    1. The surface of the food, as part of the normal course of the food's life (especially in the case of fresh cabbage and its relatives like turnips and other *Brassica* vegetables)
    2. Material from a previous round of fermentation, either similar or not to the fermentation you're attempting (for example, using yogurt to start yogurt, kombucha culture to start kombucha, or the liquid whey that separates from yogurt to start a fruit chutney)
    3. An envelope of microbes sold just for this purpose
- Next, in some cases, you may choose to stack the deck further in favor of the desired microbes by adding salt. Salt pulls moisture out of foods, creates liquid, and inhibits many undesirable microbes.
- You should consider whether or not you want the fermenting foods to be exposed to air, and package them accordingly. Sauerkraut, for example, should be protected from the air, especially early on in its fermentation, while kombucha and vinegar need air in order to brew.
- You'll need a (relatively) dark place with an appropriate temperature so that your fermentation can thrive. Sunlight is generally bad for the bacteria and yeast that you'll be courting. Ideal fermentation temperatures vary from

FERMENTATION TIME AND TEMPERATURE

FOODSTUFF	FERMENTATION TIME	FERMENTATION TEMPERATURE
Sauerkraut and Kimchi	4 days to 4 months	50°F (10°C) to 80°F (30°C)
Yogurt	12 to 24 hours	100°F (40°C) to 115°F (45°C)
Kefir	12 to 24 hours	50°F (10°C) to 100°F (40°C)
Cheese	Days to months	Varies
Hard Apple Cider	1 to 6 weeks	40°F (5°C) to 70°F (20°)
Kombucha	5 to 15 days	70°F (20°C) to 85°F (30°C)

50°F (10°C) to 110°F (43°C), depending on the food and the particular microbes involved. Some popular cool places for storing fermented foods include cellars (for pickles), caves (for cheese), and holes in the ground (for kimchi).

- Finally, you need time, so that our little friends can work their magic. The amount of time varies from one day to a couple of months or even longer.

Health Benefits of Fermentation

Some methods of food preserving affect the nutritional profiles of foods negatively. Canning, for instance, relies on heating foods to the point where all microbes are destroyed; unfortunately, heat destroys the enzymes in food that help us digest them, and diminishes or destroys many vitamins. Most other forms of preserving have some negative impact on nutrient content.

Many preservative chemicals have negative impacts on health; some of them are known carcinogens. Nonetheless, these chemicals remain in our food supply, and large-scale food processors use them because they are cheap and because they remove uncertainty from the food manufacturing process, usually by killing microbes or inhibiting enzymes.

And new techniques like irradiation, high-pressure processing, and pulsed electric field processing are not well understood; many people see serious problems with them or anticipate that we will discover serious problems with them.

By contrast, fermentation actually enhances food's nutritional value because it:

Preserves nutrients. Fermentation, because it does not involve high heat, preserves the vitamins and enzymes present in foods. In fact, beyond simply maintaining the vitamin content of raw foods, the process of fermentation can actually create new vitamins, specifically B vitamins and vitamins C and K2, as well as some types of enzymes.

Provides beneficial bacteria = a happy body. The friendly microbes that carry out the fermentation process are often themselves beneficial to humans. Plain, whole-fat yogurt, for instance, is an excellent probiotic supplement that is available in most supermarkets (the more processed kinds of yogurt aren't as healthy). Recent research is confirming what alternative practitioners have been saying for some time: Friendly bacteria in the digestive tract are crucial to a properly functioning immune system.

Helps the body digest carbohydrates. Fermentation breaks down certain types of carbohydrates that can be difficult to digest. Raw cabbage, for instance, contains polysaccharides that can lead to intestinal gas; these polysaccharides are generally broken down by fermentation, leading to a less dramatic eating experience. Likewise, some people cannot drink pasteurized milk because their bodies lack the ability to create the enzymes necessary to digest lactose (milk sugar); many of these same people have no problems with yogurt, hard cheeses, or sour cream, all of which contain significantly less lactose. (Many of these people may also be able to easily digest unpasteurized milk because it contains lactase, the enzyme required to digest lactose. This enzyme is destroyed when milk is pasteurized.)

KEY BENEFITS OF FERMENTING FOOD

Fermented food:

- preserves, sometimes enhances, vitamin content of food
- preserves, sometimes enhances, enzyme content of food
- is a healthy alternative to preservative chemical additives, some of which are toxic
- is a healthy alternative to high-tech preserving technologies, many of which are untested
- makes nutrients in foods more available to the body
- makes food less likely to cause digestive problems

"FERMENTED" VERSUS "PICKLED"

Not all pickles are fermented, and not all fermented foods are pickled. But there is a lot of overlap.

In practice, "pickled" foods are foods that have been preserved in an acid medium. Fresh vegetables can be submerged in an acidic liquid like vinegar, resulting in vegetables that are pickled, but not fermented (although vinegar itself is created via a fermentation process, so vinegar pickles actually do rely, indirectly, on fermentation). (*Note:* There are also a few pickled foods, like some pickled fish, that rely on an alkaline medium.)

Fermented vegetables generally create their own acidic liquid as a result of the fermentation, so it is fair to say that fermented vegetables are both fermented and pickled.

Finally, there are alcoholic fermented foods like wine and apple cider that are fermented but not pickled. (Although when a person is drunk, we may speak of them as being "pickled," so nothing is cut and dried—except of course foods that *have* been cut and dried.)

Stocking Your Science Lab

I tend to use mason jars (Ball jars) for fermenting just about everything. Other people use other kinds of vessels; mason jars are a pretty new thing, as far as the time scale of fermenting goes. Once you have gained some experience and confidence, I encourage you to experiment and see what works best for you!

Big strainers and colanders are much more convenient than smaller ones when washing or rinsing large vegetables. Stainless steel surfaces are better than aluminum for kitchen tools for a variety of reasons: unlike aluminum, stainless steel is nonreactive, nontoxic, and dishwasher safe.

Buy the largest chef's knife that you can comfortably wield: 8 inches (20 cm) and 10 inches (25 cm) are both good sizes. If you are cutting a big vegetable, you are much better off with a big knife, and big knives can chop more food per stroke than smaller knives can.

The Star peeler is my favorite vegetable peeler.

Rounded saucepans make stirring and cleaning easier than pans with creases; pots and pans made with aluminum cores heat more uniformly than simple stainless pans and heat up and down the sides rather than just on the bottom. (It is best to avoid having aluminum touching your food for long periods of time, especially if your food is acidic.) The Calphalon Tri-Ply (pictured on page 26) is a great medium-size saucepan.

The thermometer pictured on page 26 comes with a clip that allows you to attach it to the side of your pan in such a way that the tip of the thermometer is suspended in the liquid and does

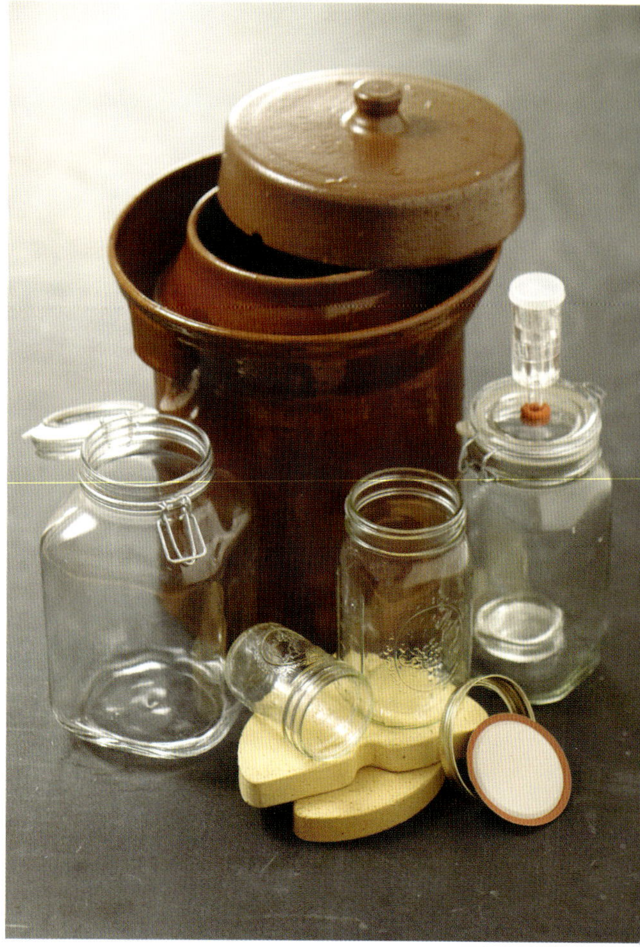

A variety of containers for fermenting. Clockwise from left: a swing-top jar; an earthenwear Harsch crock; a Pickl-It fermenting jar, with airlock; a couple of Ball jars; weights for the Harsch crock.

not touch the bottom or the sides of the saucepan. Thus, you can measure the temperature of the liquid rather than the temperature of the pan (which is likely to be hotter).

Wood is the best material for cutting boards because it is nontoxic; it does not dull your knives; and, according to some research, it is easier to clean and less likely than plastic to host malevolent microbes. (Also, it is pretty.) Do not cut directly on stainless steel, glass, or stone surfaces because these will dull your knives.

If you find yourself chopping or shredding a lot of food on a regular basis, consider investing in a food processor. It will save you a lot of time—and perhaps a shredded finger or two. If you enjoy fermenting or baking, or if you frequently find yourself cooking from recipes, a modern digital food scale is wonderful because it allows you to weigh your ingredients with great accuracy.

A 10-quart (10-L) stainless steel (not aluminum) stockpot is the smallest stockpot you should consider and may even be too small for some activities, like heating a large batch of milk for making cheese; heating a large batch of liquid in the process of brewing cider or beer; or making a large batch of stock from chicken or beef bones. You can buy carboys at specialized home-brewing stores, in person, or over the Internet; the one pictured here was originally a glass gallon cider bottle that I bought at the supermarket. An auto-siphon is another item that you are most likely to find at a home-brewing store; it allows you to pump liquid out of a large bottle without disturbing the sediment at the bottom.

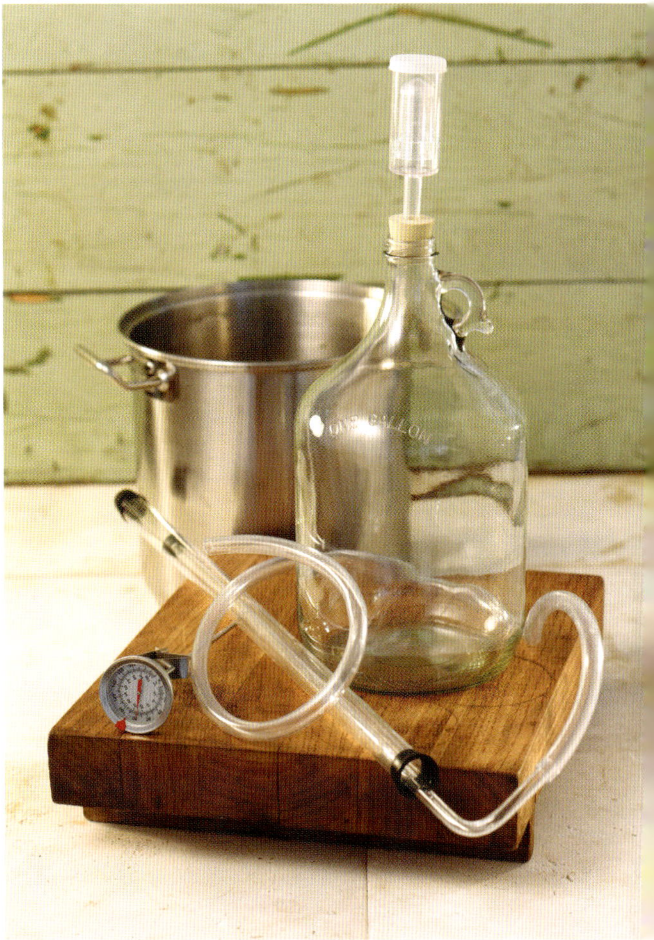

Some Cheese-making and brewing equipment. Clockwise from top left: a 10-quart (10-L) stainless steel stockpot; a 1-gallon (4-L) carboy with airlock; an auto-siphon; a thermometer; a wooden cutting board.

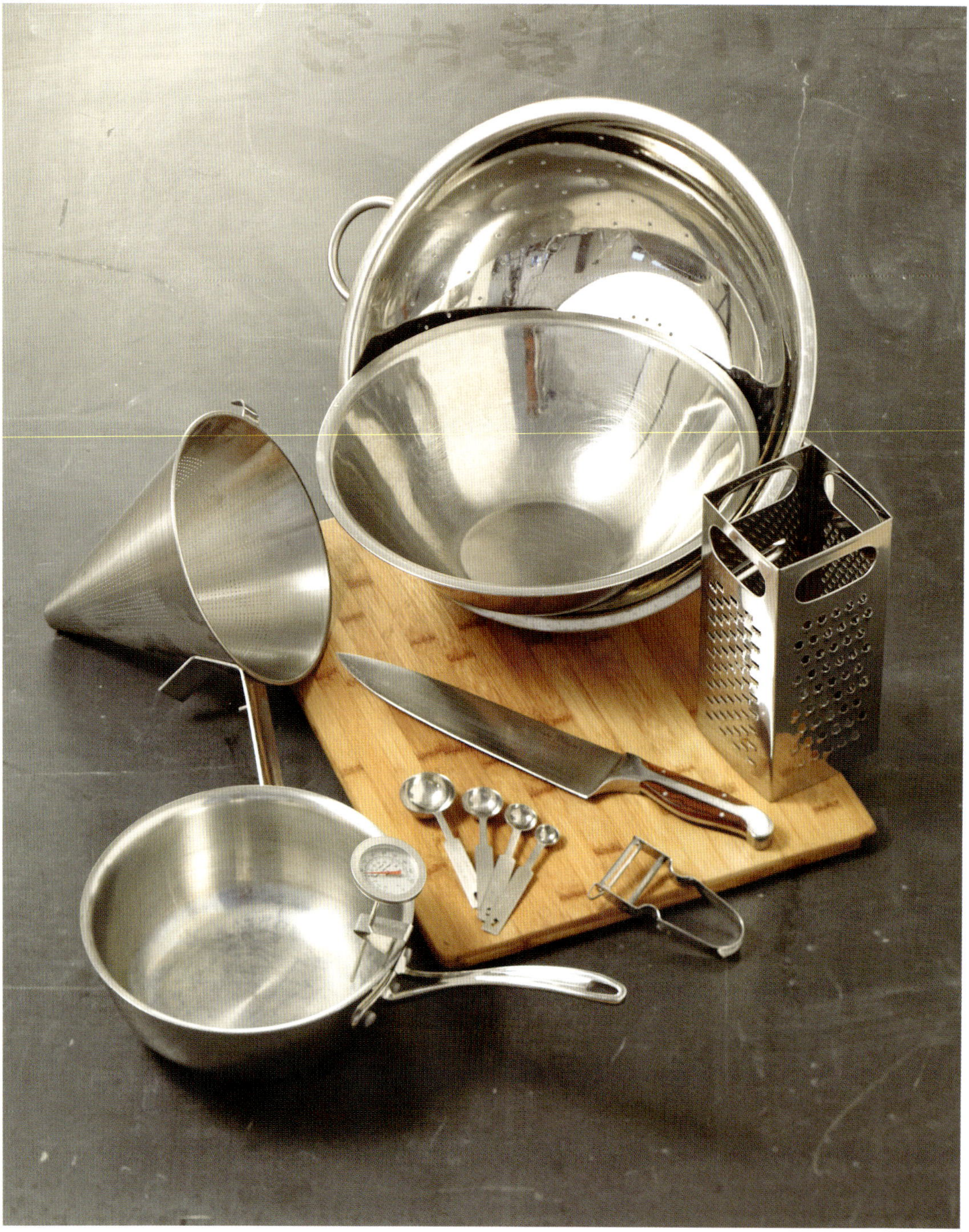

Useful kitchen tools. Clockwise from left: a conical strainer; a mixing bowl; a large colander; a box grater; a 10-inch (25-cm) chef's knife; a Star vegetable peeler; measuring spoons; a stainless steel interior, multi-ply, aluminum core, rounded saucepan; a cheese-making thermometer; a wooden cutting board.

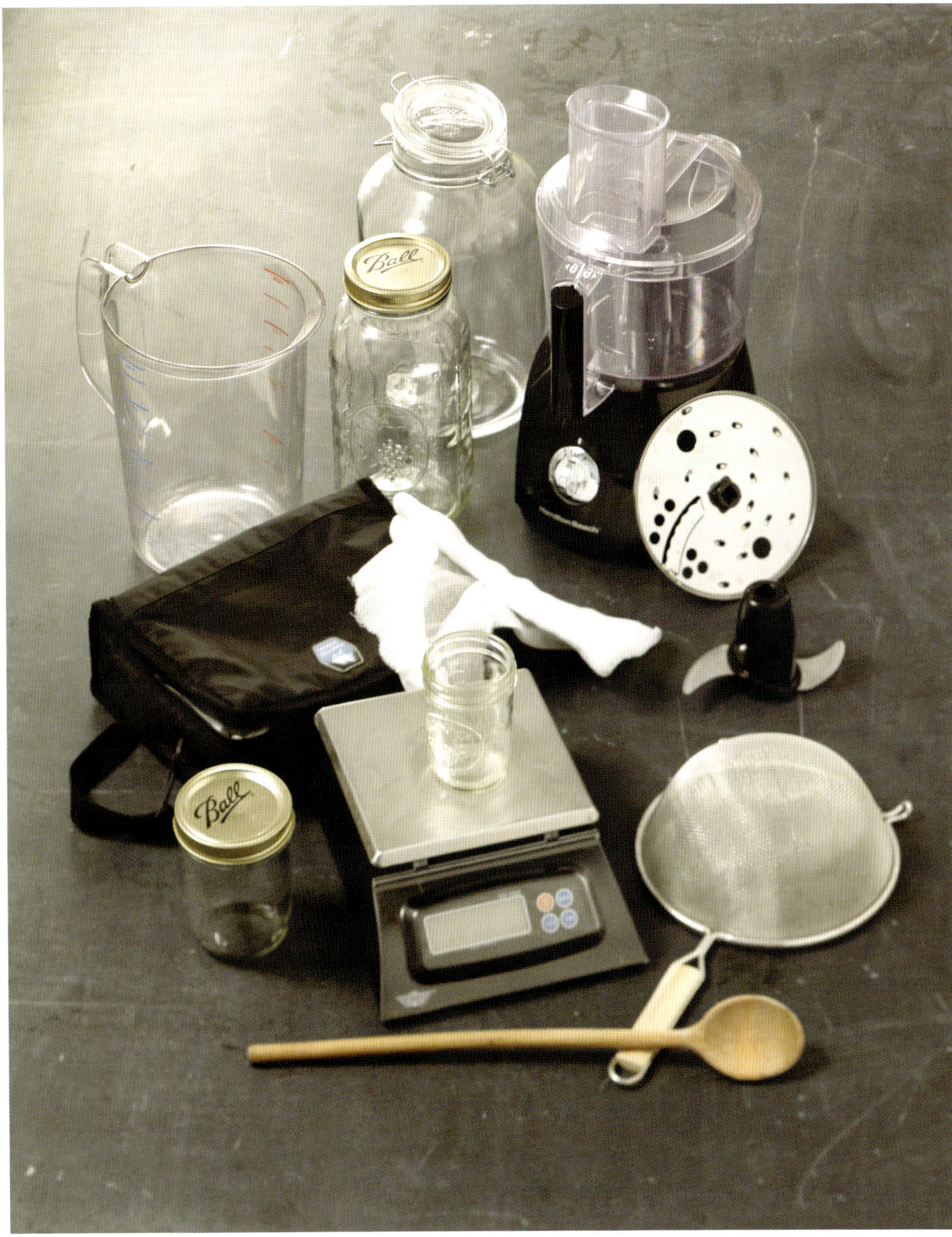

More fermentation equipment. Clockwise from left: an insulated lunch bag (useful for making yogurt); a gallon (4L) pitcher; various Ball and swing-top jars; a food processor, with slicer wheel; a strainer; a wooden spoon; a digital food scale; some cheesecloth.

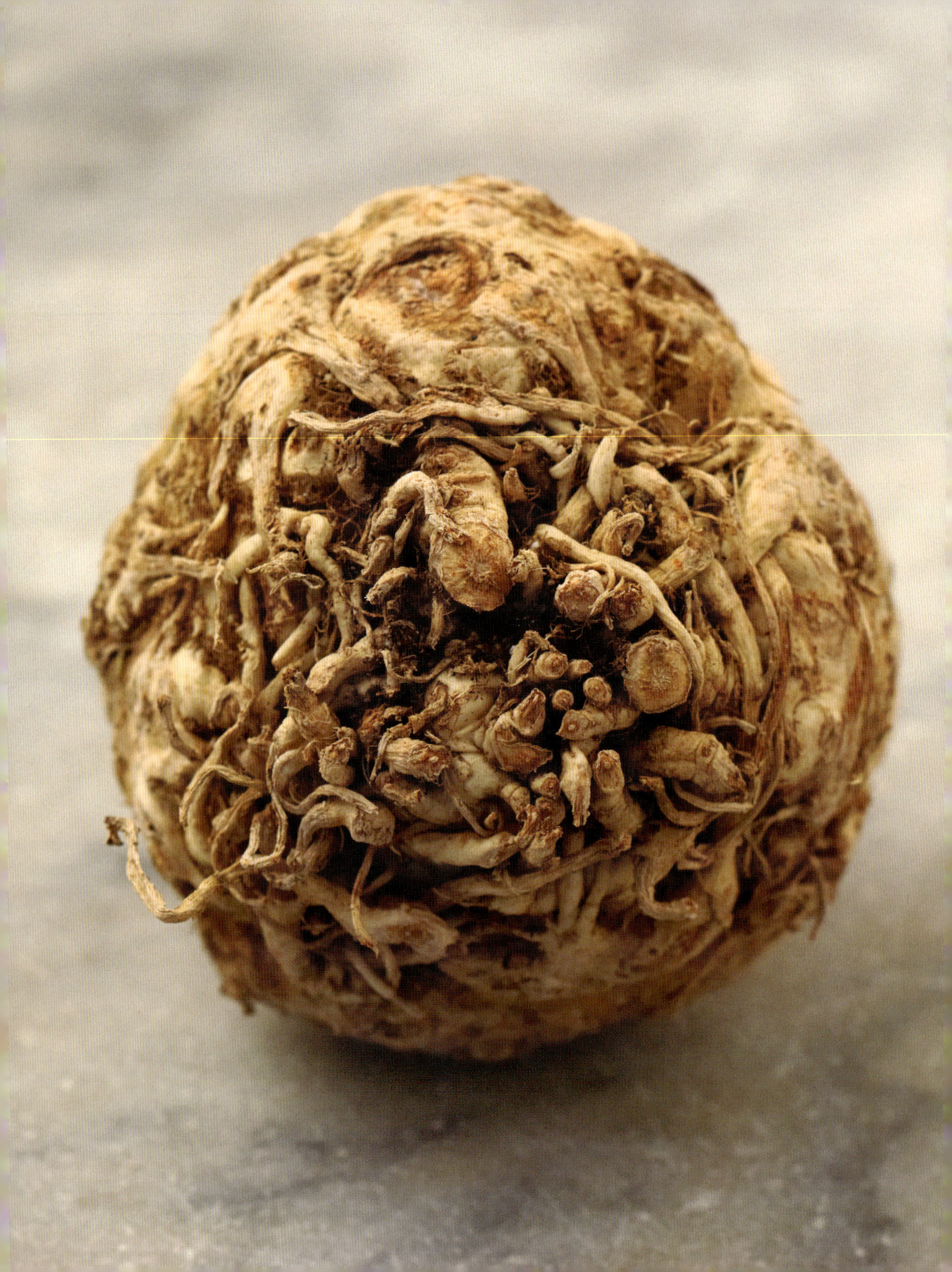

CHAPTER 2

Know Your Ingredients

Choosing the best ingredients is key to having your creations turn out as delicious and nutritious as possible.

Many factors help determine what the "best" ingredients are. Freshness is one: Generally, the fresher your ingredients, the better the result. This often means choosing food produced locally and in season. Production method is another: Food produced with a minimum of industrial inputs will taste better and be better for you. Organic can be helpful, but it is not the whole story. The genetics of the food itself are important: Genetically modified foods are recent creations, and there are already signs that they are not at all the same as their traditional counterparts. Insufficient testing was done before they were unleashed on the public, so unless you would like to be part of the ongoing test, they are best avoided.

For nonanimal, nonvegetable ingredients, chemical purity is a factor. If a recipe calls for water, then the purer the water, the better. Chlorine, for instance, is found in much of the municipal water supply and should be removed, both because it is bad for you and because it can get in the way of fermentation. Likewise, much of the salt sold at the supermarket contains chemicals that are added to prevent it from clumping, or for other reasons; unfortunately, these chemicals can taste bad, be unhealthy, or, worst of all, impede your fermentation!

The best way to be certain about the provenance and purity of your ingredients is to make your food from scratch when possible. This is one of the greatest things you can do for yourself, for your community, and for your family.

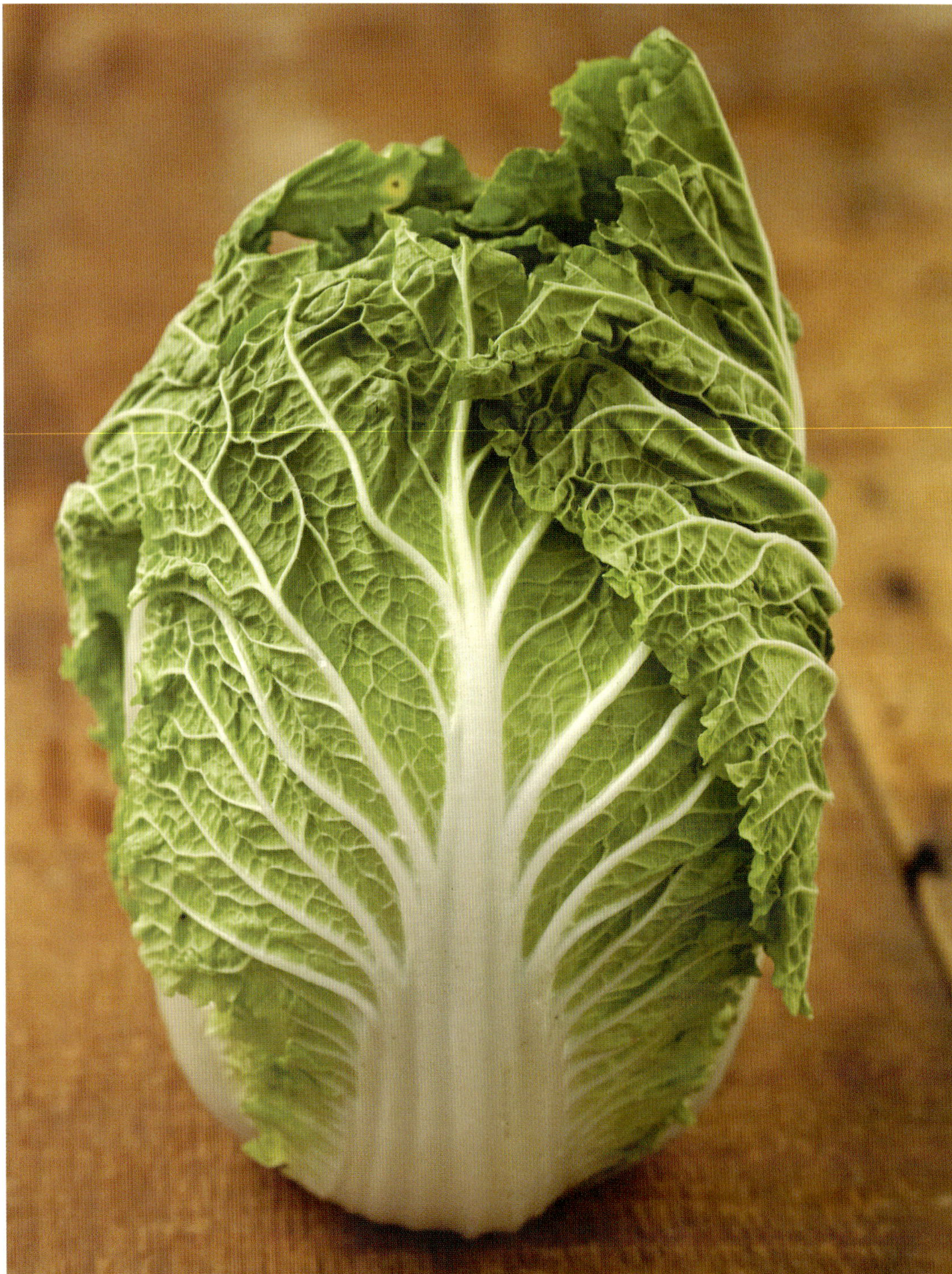

Fresh, organic Napa cabbage, fit to be fermented.

The Freshness Factor

Fresher ingredients are generally better. Here's why.

- Raw food naturally contains enzymes. From the moment vegetables are picked, these enzymes start to break them down and make them mushy. (The same thing happens with meat, although some amount of breakdown can actually improve meat.)
- Certain flavors and vitamins in food decay over time when exposed to heat, light, and air.
- As food sits around, microbes and other things start nibbling on it. If we don't take precautions, bacteria, molds, fungi, yeasts, insects, rodents, bears, and so on can eat our food, or render it unsafe for human consumption.

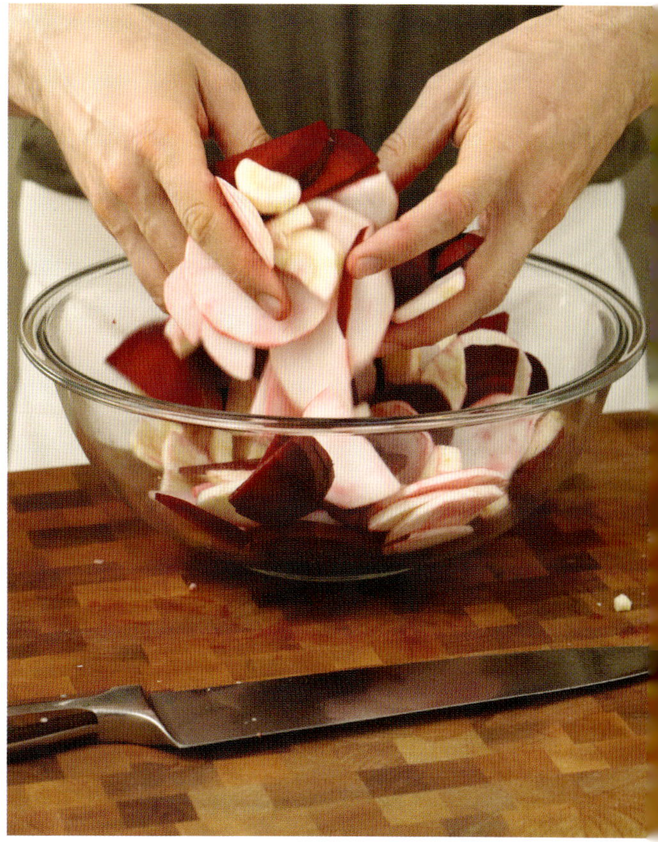

Sliced red beets and turnips are combined for a late-spring batch of brined vegetables.

Buying Local and In Season

When you buy vegetables at a farmers' market, you can ask the vendor when the vegetables were picked, where they were grown, what farming methods were used, and so on.

When you buy vegetables at a supermarket, you may not be able to get this information—and the vegetables will probably have been sitting around longer, especially if they came from far away. You can usually find out what country the vegetables are from, but often not much more.

Buying Organic

In the United States, products labeled "Organic," "USDA Organic," or "100% Organic" are legally required to have been produced in particular ways. Only specific types of fertilizers, pesticides, and herbicides can be used, and producers must pay fees to qualified certification agencies.

Outside the United States, countries, unions, and jurisdictions have similar labeling laws. For instance, any products marked with the EU organic logo are subject to certain requirements regarding inputs, inspections, and certifications.

Before "organic" acquired legal meanings, it was used colloquially to describe food produced in a "natural" way, without industrially produced treatments or soil amendments.

The problem with the old, informal system was that it was not specific, was not regulated, and was a matter of trust. The problem with the new, official system is that small producers may not be able to pay the certification fees without financial hardship. Also, the new system creates a simple dichotomy—organic versus nonorganic—that can

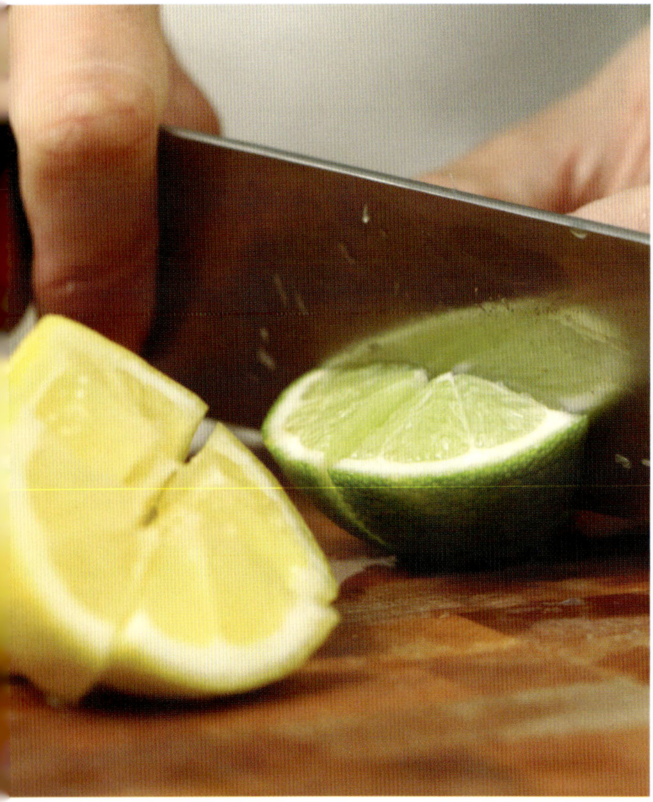

Citrus fruit is a very region-specific crop, and close conversations with the grower before buying may not be an option.

mask some of the food's other characteristics that may also be important, such as locality, seasonality, and time to market.

Having said all of this, it is still true that in a super-market, organic is usually better than nonorganic.

Buying organic vegetables and fruit is particularly important when:

- you plan to eat the rind, peel, skin, or outermost portions of the food (as you might with apples, grapes, soft fruit, or citrus);
- you are buying particular types of food that either tend to get a lot of pesticides applied to them or tend to absorb pesticides (such as bell peppers, celery, collard greens, and apples);
- some of your eaters are sick, old, or have weakened or sensitive immune systems.

The Environmental Working Group publishes a "Shopper's Guide to Pesticides in Produce," which can be helpful in assessing some of the potential risks of non-organic fruit and vegetables.

When you are able to talk to a food producer—at a farmers' market, for instance—you can have a longer conversation about farming practices, why something may or may not be certified organic, why the producer made specific decisions, and so on. "Certified organic" does not always mean "more natural," particularly in the case of meat, eggs, and dairy. For example, certified organic eggs can be laid by chickens who practically never go outside and never eat the bugs and worms that they need for optimal health, while small, local farms may produce eggs that are more nutritious, fresher, and better in almost every way, but are not certified organic.

Similarly, organic vegetables produced and processed on a large scale can have more opportunity to become contaminated during picking, processing, packing, and shipping than vegetables from a small local farm.

Genetically Modified

Genetically modified organisms (GMOs) are those whose DNA has been modified in a laboratory. DNA is the blueprint for all living things. By splicing in pieces of DNA from different species, often very different ones, scientists aim to engineer the characteristics of a particular genetically modified plant or animal. For instance, a significant fraction of corn sold in the United States today contains DNA from a species of bacteria named *Bacillus thuringiensis*;

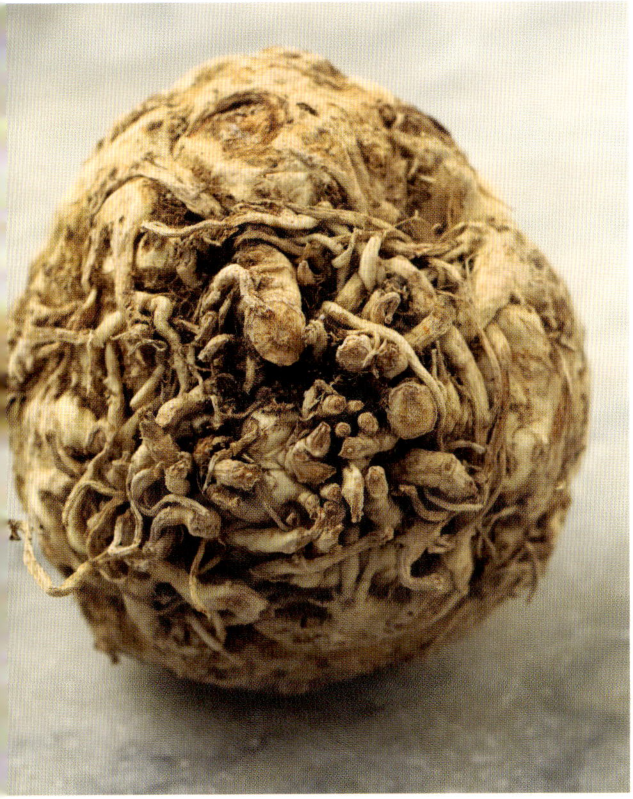

Celery root

this alteration makes the corn toxic to certain pests. The supposed advantage of the modification is that it decreases the "need" for spraying pesticides on this crop.

Some scientists, including of course those working for the companies that develop and sell GMO technology, claim that eating genetically modified (GM) food is safe. Other scientists believe that GM food is dangerous and has contributed to a variety of singularly modern problems, including allergies, autoimmune diseases, decline of bee populations, and so on. They also point out that the GM food regulatory approval process is far too short and maintain that because of this, we can't properly assess the long-term effects of GM foods on human, animal, or plant populations, or on the ecosystem as a whole.

It may be prudent to avoid genetically modified foods until we see which side wins this debate. At the very least, you might consider evaluating the competing arguments yourself before making a decision about whether or not you want to eat GM foods—or really, continue eating them, because if you haven't been paying *very* close attention, you've been eating them for years.

If you decide to avoid GM foods, the next step is to identify which foods have been genetically modified.

- In many countries, including most of Europe and Russia, GM foods are required to be labeled as such.
- The United States has no requirement for specific labeling of GM foods, but basic food items that are certified organic are guaranteed not to be genetically modified. Processed foods labeled "100% organic" are guaranteed not to contain GM ingredients—but if they are merely labeled "organic," they *may* contain some percentage of ingredients derived from GM foods.
- The variety of GM foods approved for human consumption changes from year to year, as do surrounding regulations.

Up-to-date information about GM foods, including arguments for and against, can be found in scientific journal articles. But the most significant new findings get summarized and discussed on the Internet immediately; that's where the public dialogue occurs, and it's probably the best place to find the latest news.

Water

Some fermentation recipes call for the use of water or brine. Municipal tap water can contain varying amounts of chlorine and/or a related chemical called chloramine. These are added by the water authorities to prevent the propagation of microbes of various sorts. Chlorine and chloramine do this very well. The problem is that successful fermentation depends on the propagation of microbes! So for fermenting purposes, it is good to remove as much chlorine and chloramine as possible from the water.

There are various ways to try to remove chlorine and chloramine from water. These work to varying degrees.

- Leave the water out in an open container for 12 to 24 hours. This allows chlorine to come out of solution with the water and escape into the air. It works less well with chloramine.
- Boil the water for a couple of minutes and allow it to cool. This forces chlorine gas to boil away.
- Use a carbon water filter (pitcher filter, faucet filter, or under-sink filter).
- Use a reverse osmosis filter. These are available at most home improvement stores or for purchase online.

Reverse osmosis filters are generally the best solution when they're practical because they address some other potential problems with your water. For example, municipal water sometimes contains fluoride, fertilizer and pesticide residues, pharmaceutical residues, volatile organic compounds, heavy metals, and, in some places, biological threats like amoebas and protozoa. You do not want to consume any of these, either.

In most places, if you ask them for it, your water company will provide you with a written analysis of your local water.

Salt

Sea salt, salt from dried lake beds, and Himalayan salt are good choices. They naturally contain trace minerals that are important for your health. Expect them to be gray or pink, not quite white. (Note that concern has been raised recently about the microplastic content in sea salt. Research this if you are curious.)

If you can't get one of these, it is too expensive in a particular context, or you are making a big batch of brine that will not be consumed directly, then look for salt that contains only salt as an ingredient! Check the label. Kosher salt is often a good choice (but read the ingredients list).

Table salt often contains additives to prevent clumping. It may also contain additives to address some public health need, such as iodine to prevent goiter. These additives can add unpleasant tastes to foods and can impede your fermentation projects.

Getting Real about Food

Until a hundred or so years ago, most people in most parts of the world spent significant time pondering food, procuring food from nearby or known sources, and preparing food at home. Recently, we have spent less and less time on food. Over the course of the past century, we've gone from eating 98 percent of meals in our homes to 50 percent. And the food that we eat in our homes nowadays often comes in the form of frozen meals, "convenience" foods, soda, chips, and food-like substances that defy categorization. People in rich countries are not alone in this—the people of poorer countries have become eager consumers of soda, chips, and fast food and are squarely in the crosshairs of global food marketers.

Most snack foods, prepared foods, and restaurant foods in the United States, and in much of the world, are industrially produced. They are generally not environmentally sound because of the manufacture, processing, packaging, and transportation involved in their creation and delivery. Neither are they nutritionally sound: Their signature ingredients—high-fructose corn syrup, processed vegetable oils, white flour, flavoring chemicals, preservative chemicals, and so on—are used because they are cheap, addictive, and shelf stable, not because they are wholesome or nutritious in any way. In fact, many of these ingredients are harmful to us.

The best way for us to reverse this trend is simply to pay more attention to food. Every choice we make about food has an impact on the world. It also has an impact on us, for what we're putting into our bodies at that moment, for the habits we're forming for ourselves, and for the example that we're setting for others around us. Because you are reading this book, it's likely that you think about food more than most of the people you know—and it's likely that some of them look to you for guidance and inspiration about what and how to eat. (Some of them may have no choice!)

This is why it is important for us to make our own food.

On a broader level, thinking about food in a deep way can lead us to examine the politics and economics of food production and distribution. These issues are intertwined with some of the biggest problems of the day. It is easy to imagine how food politics might be related to famine and malnutrition, for instance. But there are many other problems in which food systems play a large role:

- chronic disease because of the way that diet affects health
- resource wars: today oil, soon water, because industrial food production relies on oil for fertilization, treatment, harvesting, and transportation, and on water for irrigation
- fragile financial markets and the complexities of globalization because the world is now one big, uneven market for commodity food
- use and misuse of technologies, including pesticides and weed killers, antibiotics, and genetically modified organisms

And so on.

Making Your Own Food

Every time you contemplate your next meal, you face choices.

Where: Do I eat at home or at a restaurant? When I'm eating with family or friends, do we make food and eat in our homes, or do we go out?

How: Do I cook from scratch, completely or partially, or do I buy food that has been prepared ahead of time by someone else, using processes and ingredients that may or may not be what I would have preferred or expected?

What: Do I get my ingredients as directly as possible from their producers, or do I pay a commercial food aggregator (often a "supermarket") for the convenience of one-stop shopping?

Another consideration for most people is expense. How much does food cost where you live? How much of your income are you willing or able to spend on it? How much more would you spend to get food that tasted better? Or on food that could potentially decrease your medical bills? Or for food that you thought was better for the world?

These are choices you make based on what is important to you.

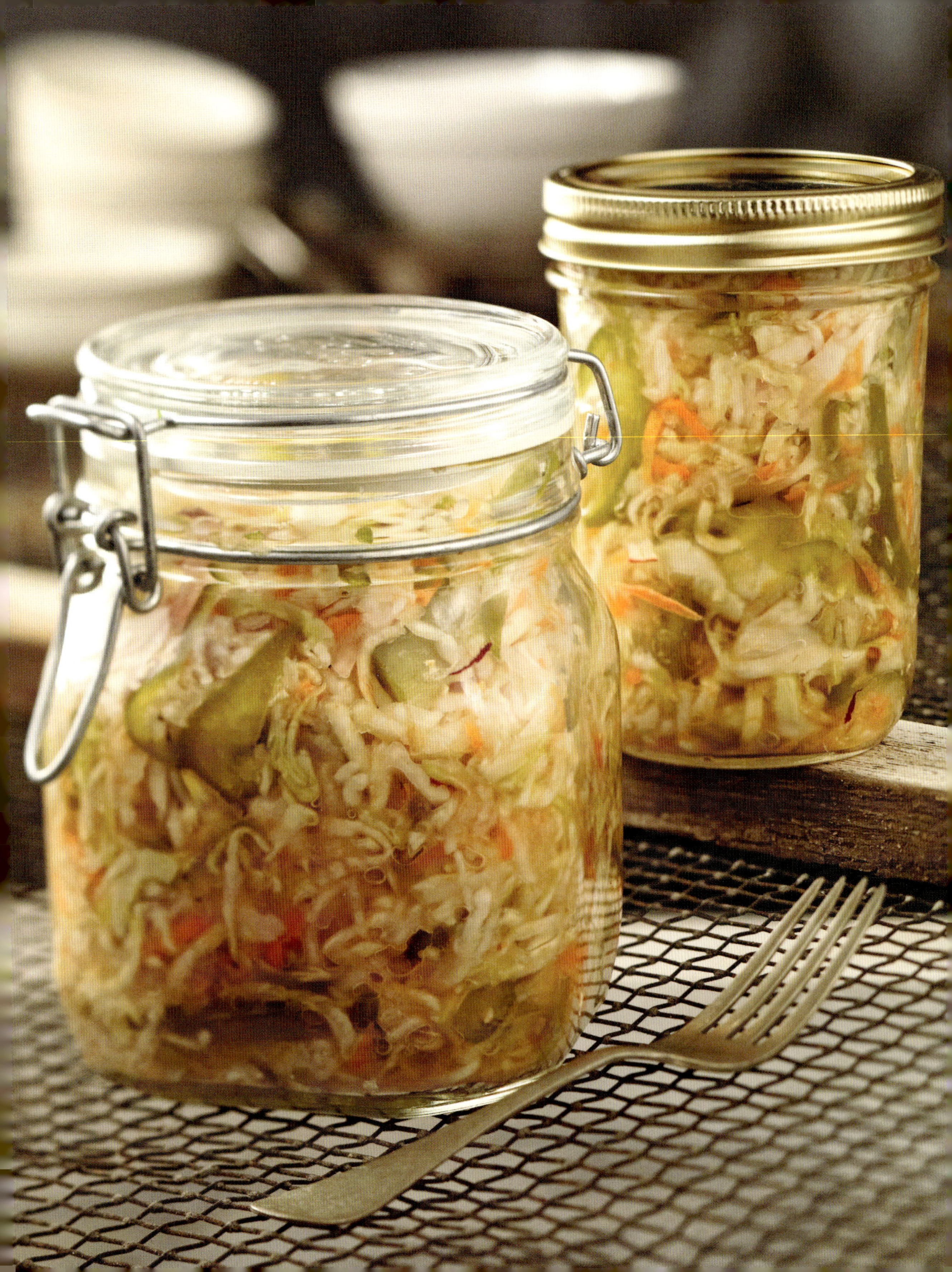

CHAPTER 3

Sauerkraut and Lacto-Fermented Vegetables

Sauerkraut is a food whose salient ingredient is lacto-fermented cabbage—green, red, savoy, napa, or otherwise.

Sauerkraut has a colorful history. It has existed in one form or another, by one name or another, for at least several thousand years. Evidence has been found of sauerkraut in the diets of the workers building the Great Wall of China; Pliny wrote of sauerkraut in ancient Rome; fermented cabbage has been a mainstay of cold-weather European diets since at least the Middle Ages; and sailors have carried it on ships to ward off scurvy, which it can do because of its high vitamin C content.

As a first fermentation project, sauerkraut is ideal. It is simple and relatively quick to make, has a high success rate, and is delicious. Sauerkraut can be eaten on its own, of course, but it can also be eaten on a sandwich, in a soup or stew, with meat or fish, with eggs, in a dumpling, or however you like.

Its appeal is international. Kimchi—a sauerkraut relative that includes ginger, garlic, onions, and, often, spicy red pepper and other seasonings—is the uncontested national dish of Korea. It is often eaten for three meals a day, as a side dish, and also in stews, stir-fries, fried rice, soup, and so on. *Choucroute garnie*, which I think of as "the queen of sauerkraut dishes," is a casserole of pork, sausages, potatoes, juniper berries, Riesling, and, of course, sauerkraut that is a favorite in the Alsace region of France.

Sauerkraut is the archetype of fermented vegetables. But cabbage is not the only vegetable that can be fermented. You can ferment other vegetables along with cabbage without changing the proportion of vegetable to salt. You can ferment a vegetable mix containing little or no cabbage. You can throw in some fruit. And there are even ways to ferment vegetables with little or no salt.

WHY YOU MUST READ ABOUT SAUERKRAUT

Even if you don't like sauerkraut, please read about it anyway. The issues that come up while making sauerkraut are the same issues that come up while making other fermented vegetables and fruits. Thus, sauerkraut is a great jumping-off point and an excellent template for further fermenting adventures. And maybe if you made your own sauerkraut you would like it!

Important parts of the sauerkraut-making process that apply to other fermenting projects include the following:

- selecting raw materials and equipment
- using a knife and cutting board
- measuring and weighing ingredients
- mixing the vegetables with salt
- deciding whether to add a fermentation starter
- packing the product tightly in a fermenting jar
- testing it for readiness

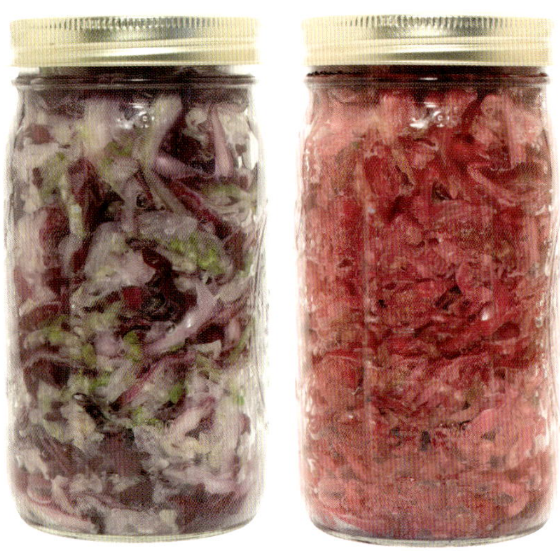

Red cabbage sauerkraut at 5 days (left) and at 10 days (right)

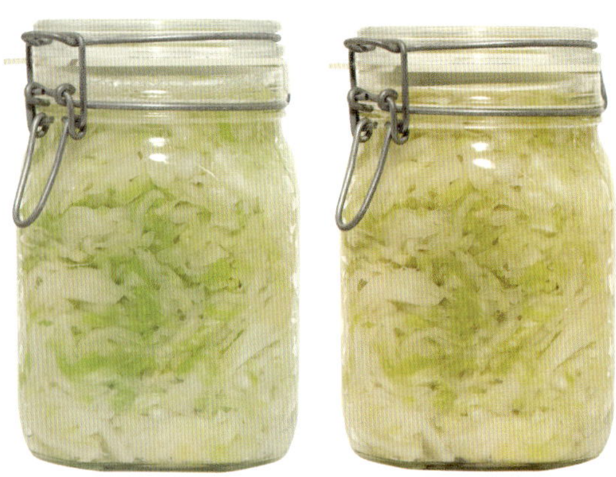

Green cabbage sauerkraut at 5 days (left) and at 10 days (right)

Basic Sauerkraut

PREP TIME: 10 MINUTES • TOTAL TIME: 4 DAYS–4 WEEKS

In its basic form, sauerkraut contains only two ingredients: cabbage and salt. The recipe can be varied by adding other vegetables or seasonings. By eating it young or letting it ferment for a longer time, you can choose between crunchy, slightly sour cabbage; epic, Wagnerian sauerkraut; or anything in between.

INGREDIENTS

2 pounds (1 kg) cabbage (green and red cabbage work best for this simple sauerkraut recipe)

4 teaspoons (20 g) sea salt

If your cabbage is not exactly 2 pounds (1 kg), use approximately 2 teaspoons (10 g) of sea salt per pound (0.5 kg) of cabbage. Alternatively, you can use 2 percent salt by weight.

For best results, weigh your cabbage *after* you have removed its outer leaves and core.

EQUIPMENT

Large cutting board (wood is ideal)

Large knife (a chef's knife is ideal)

Large mixing bowl

1-quart (1-L) mason jar, or similar glass jar with a tight-fitting lid

—

Yield: 1 quart (1 L)

PREPARATION

1. Peel off the outer leaves of the cabbage and discard them (a). (*Note:* This is particularly important if your cabbage is not organically grown. For more on choosing ingredients, see chapter 2.)

2. If you are working with a whole cabbage, cut it in half, from the south pole to the north pole (b).

3. Cut each half once more, along the north-south axis, so that the whole cabbage is now in four pieces (c).

4. *Optional:* Remove some of the core of the cabbage by cutting diagonally into each quarter (d).

continued

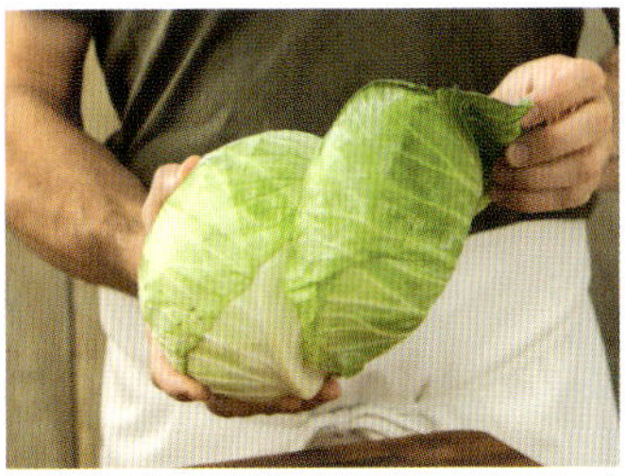

a

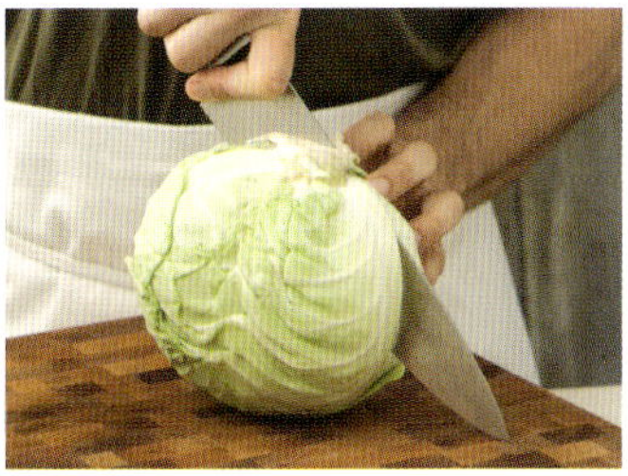

b

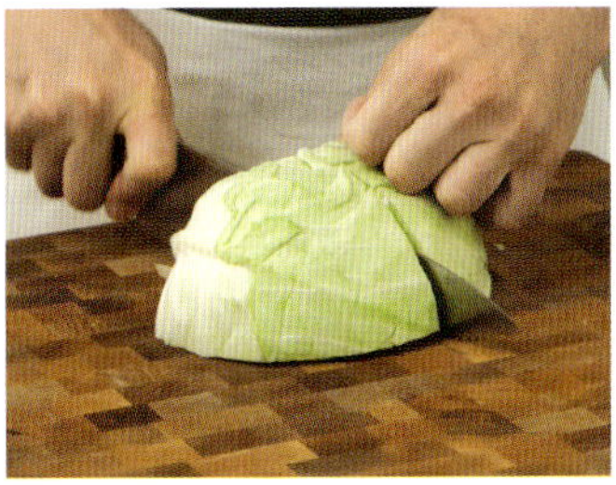

c

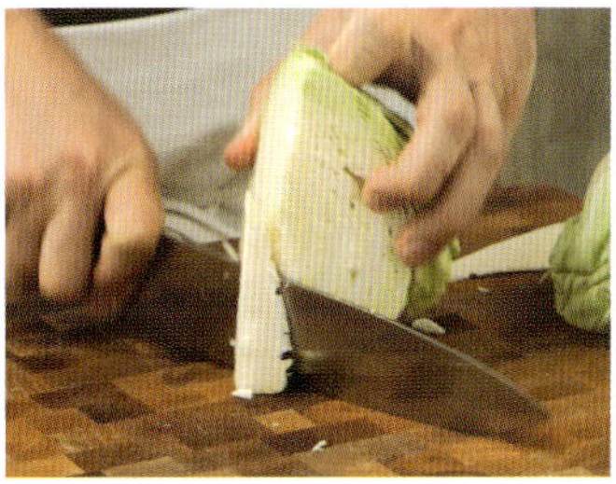

d

Basic Sauerkraut *(continued)*

5. With its south pole facing you, lay a quarter of the cabbage on your cutting board, and slice it as finely or as coarsely as you like (e). More finely cut cabbage will ferment more quickly and will become a softer kraut. Coarser cut cabbage will lead to a crunchier product. Be careful of your fingers!

6. When it becomes awkward to slice, turn or flip the cabbage quarter in whatever way is convenient to make it more stable on the cutting board and easier to cut.

7. If you prefer, use a food processor with a "slice" wheel to shred your cabbage (f). You could also use a deli-style meat slicer, a box grater, or a purpose-built *Krauthobel.*

8. Slice the rest of the cabbage in this manner. When you are done, put it all in the mixing bowl and add the salt (g).

9. With clean hands, *firmly* massage the mixture of cabbage and salt until you are able to squeeze liquid out of the cabbage (h). Depending on how fresh the cabbage is, how much cabbage you have, and how hard you are squeezing, this may take anywhere from 1 to 10 minutes. You will develop a feel for it after you have done it a few times.

10. Pack the mixture into a jar or jars (i). Using an appropriately sized implement, such as a small jar or potato masher, push down as hard as you can to get rid of as many air bubbles as possible, so that the liquid rises above the top of the cabbage. Ensure that there is at least 1 inch (2.5 cm) of space between the top of the cabbage and the mouth of the jar, because the cabbage will expand as it ferments.

> *For each pound (0.5 kg) of cabbage you use, you will need a bit more than 16 ounces (500 ml) of jar capacity. Depending on the size of your jars, you can use a small jar to help pack the sauerkraut into the bigger jars.*

11. Close the lid of the jar finger-tight and place it in a cool, dark place, if possible (between 50°F and 75°F [10°C and 25°C]).

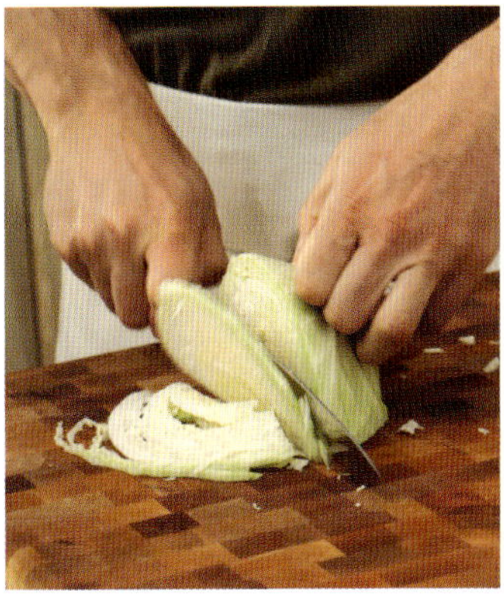

e

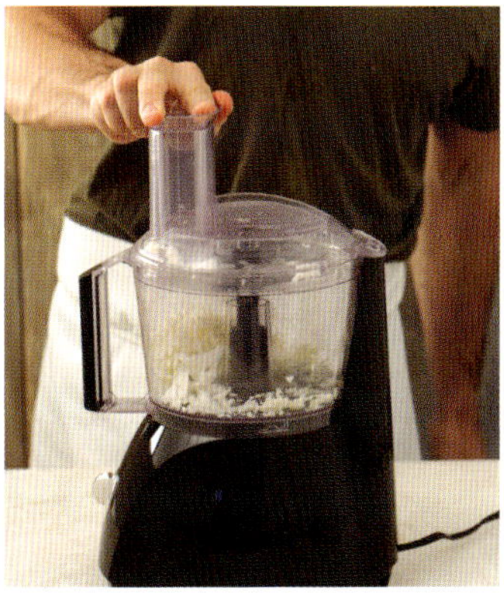

f (optional)

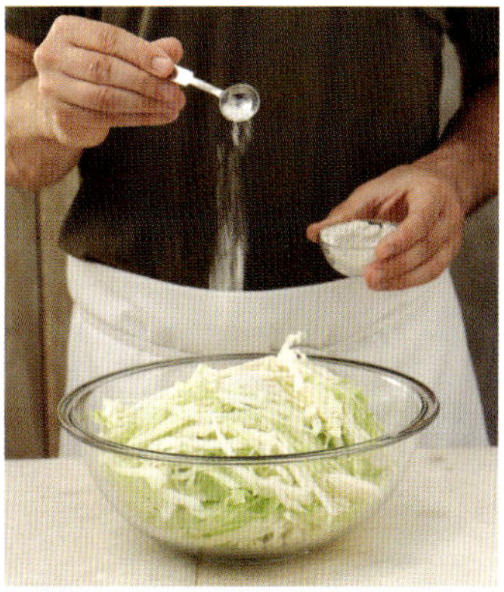

g

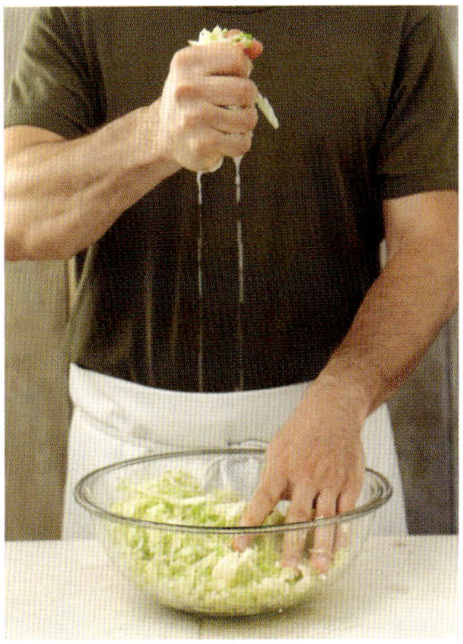

h

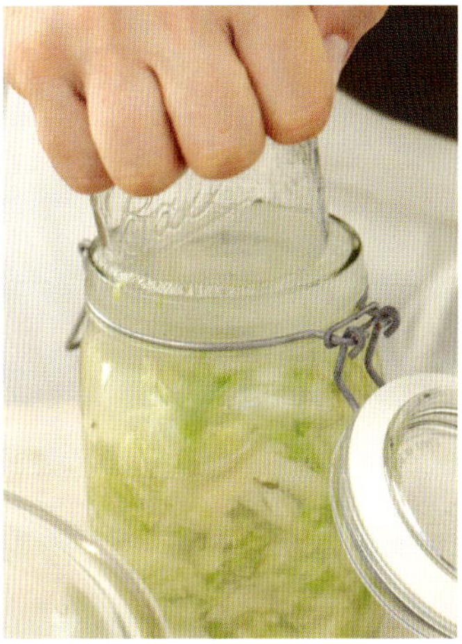

i

FERMENTATION PROCESS

After you finish canning your sauerkraut, check on it every day or two. Open the jar, smell it, taste it with a clean fork, and pack the sauerkraut back down until the liquid rises above it. After a few days, it should get bubbly. After a few more days, it should start to smell and taste sour.

You can eat it any time you want, or you can put it the refrigerator to arrest its progress. Young sauerkraut is crunchier; older sauerkraut has a stronger flavor.

For maximum digestive and nutritive benefits, eat your sauerkraut raw (i.e., do not heat it beyond about 115°F [46°C]). However, if digestive and nutritive benefits are not your main goals, there's no shame in cooking your sauerkraut. In fact, old sauerkraut that has become soggy and very sour may taste best cooked.

Which Vegetables (and/or Fruit) Should I Use?

Some vegetables, like cabbage, ferment easily, while others require extra attention, guidance, and/or coercion.

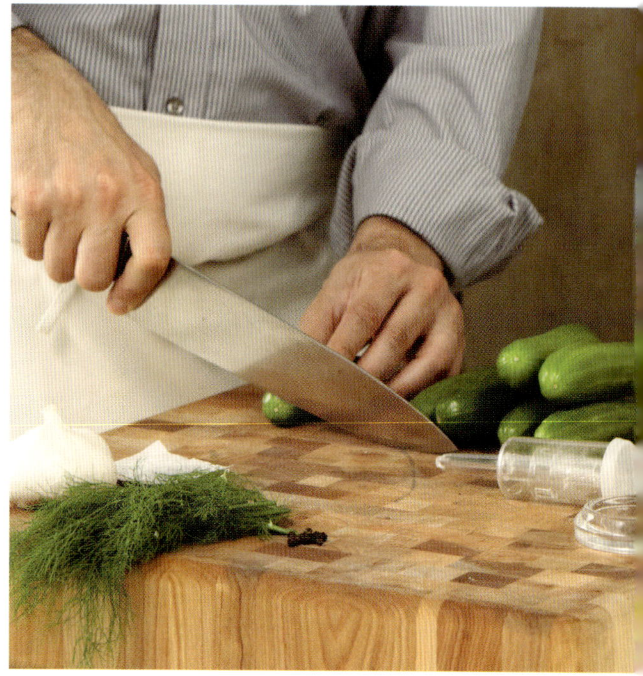

Good Fermenters

The best fermenting vegetables are from the family *Brassicaceae*, also known as cruciferous vegetables. These include cabbage, turnips, kohlrabi, and radishes. They have a firm texture and relatively low sugar content.

Okay Fermenters

Vegetables like onions, carrots, and celery root do well when mingled with good fermenters. If you seek to ferment them on their own, you might want to use a starter (see next page).

Temperamental Fermenters

When most people think of pickles and pickling, they think of cucumbers. Interestingly, fermenting cucumbers can be tricky. Fermented cucumbers can succumb to "hollow pickle syndrome," wherein the inside of the pickle disintegrates; this is often accompanied by general softness of the pickle. Likewise, summer squashes and bell peppers can become disconcertingly soft (ripe bell peppers are trickier than green ones). These problems come from the work of enzymes on the relatively weak physical structure of these vegetables.

With vegetables that don't ferment very well, consider using a starter, using a generous concentration of salt, and even seeking additional insurance (see page 44). Cutting off the blossom ends of these vegetables mitigates some of the enzyme issues, too (see chapter 1).

Beets, parsnips, apples, pears, and other sweet fruit, because of their higher sugar content, tend to attract yeasts that can cause the fermentation to veer off in the direction of alcohol generation. This is great if you are trying to make an alcoholic beverage, but if you are trying to make lacto-fermented vegetables and fruit, it is not what you want. If you combine these sweet vegetables and fruits with well-behaved ones like cabbage and turnips, you will generally get the results you expect (i.e., lacto-fermentation). Sweet vegetables and fruit can be lacto-fermented on their own with the use of a starter.

Vegetables to Avoid

Raw potatoes contain compounds called glycoalkaloids, which are neurotoxic (poisonous to your brain and your nervous system). So potatoes are not good candidates for raw fermenting—or raw anything, for that matter.

TROUBLESHOOTING: FERMENTATION GONE WRONG

What can go wrong with a vegetable ferment, and how can I fix it?

If it tastes too salty: Add water judiciously, stir the whole thing up, possibly drain out some of the liquid, and give everything some time to rebalance.

If the top of the batch of vegetables has dried up: It may be possible to revive the batch by stirring it up (submerging the dry part at the top), and then adding some water or brine.

If the vegetables have become too soft or mushy: You cannot reverse this, but if they are just a little soft or mushy, they may be used in a soup or a stew, where vegetables go to become soft and mushy anyway. They are best added at the last minute, or even after the dish has started to cool, so that they don't cook for a long time and become even more soft and mushy, and also so that their beneficial microbes and nutrients aren't all destroyed by heat.

If they became too soft sooner than you hoped, there are measures you can take in the future to improve the texture. These measures include using more salt, using a starter, or adding something else, like grape leaves, for the specific purpose of decreasing mushiness (see page 44 for more on fermenting "insurance").

If the vegetables have become slimy, if there is visible fuzz or significant mold growing on top, or if they smell bad or of alcohol: This indicates that the fermentation did not go as planned, probably having been hijacked by molds or yeasts or both. It won't taste good, it won't have good texture, and eating it could be risky. Send it to the compost heap!

Do I Need to Peel Everything Beforehand?

Organic whole vegetables may be peeled or not, as you like. If not peeled, they can be scrubbed clean with a vegetable brush; soap is not needed. Nonorganic vegetables should always be peeled to get rid of as much of the pesticide residue as possible; nonorganic leafy vegetables should have their outer leaves removed.

Which Starter Should I Use, If Any?

A starter is a collection of microbes that you add to your food to encourage it to ferment in the way that you want.

Fermentation projects based on well-behaved fermenters and salt do not generally require a starter because they naturally tend to attract the right sorts of microbes. Projects based on more troublesome vegetables and fruits, or lower than usual amounts of salt, on the other hand, can benefit from a nudge (or a shove) in the right direction.

You have three options (at least) for fermented vegetable starters:

Liquid from a previous batch of homemade sauerkraut or other fermented vegetables (not too young and not too old—say, between 4 days and 4 weeks): This starter is easy to make, and its freshness is known. It tends to impart a fermented vegetable flavor when added; in many cases (when making fermented vegetables, for instance), this is not a problem. Some have expressed concern that using fermented vegetable liquid hijacks the typical progression of lacto-fermentation microbes. Try it for yourself and see what you think.

Live dairy whey from yogurt, kefir, or clabbered raw milk (the younger the better): This is a good, powerful starter that is easy to make. To make yogurt whey, put yogurt in cheesecloth; the liquid that drips out is whey. (See recipe on page 74.) Whey can impart a slight milky taste or texture, even when strained carefully. Because it is a dairy product, vegans, kosher eaters, and those with sensitivity to casein or acute sensitivity to lactose should be aware of this.

Purpose-made vegetable fermentation starter culture: Powdered starter cultures are sold in envelopes. They should be kept cool until used, and it is important to pay attention to their expiration dates. A purpose-made starter, assuming it has been transported and stored properly, can produce excellent, consistent results without any stray flavors. However, these starters do cost money, and purists might object to using these packaged goods. They sometimes contain dairy.

Do I Want Additional Fermenting Insurance?

As I noted previously, cucumber pickles and summer squash have a tendency to digest themselves. (This self-digestion is called autolysis.) Even a recipe that works most of the time, in most places, might not turn out as you had hoped, depending on the ingredients you are using, the temperature and humidity, the ambient bacteria where you are, or just plain bad luck.

Beyond using a starter, there are a few things you can do to further improve your odds of success, especially with cucumbers:

- You can add some vinegar to immediately increase acidity. Boiled red wine vinegar and cider vinegar are good options because of the tannins they contain (see the next item); distilled white vinegar works well, too. Raw wine or cider vinegar may not work as well because they contain their own set of microbes that are not really the ones you want and that could potentially take over your pickles. If you'd like to use wine or cider vinegar, boil it first, and then let it cool.
- For centuries, people have been adding grape leaves, oak leaves, bay leaves, and other tannic leaves to cucumber pickles in order to keep them crunchy. As we now know, tannins inhibit cucumbers' naturally occurring pectinase and cellulase enzymes that would otherwise cause the cucumbers to digest themselves. Grape skins contain tannins, too, so red wine vinegar can be a double help. Other good sources of tannins include apple cider vinegar, cloves, tarragon, cumin, thyme, vanilla, and cinnamon—some of which are found in pickling spice mixes (I don't think this is a coincidence). Finally, black tea, loose or in tea bags, contains tannins and can give your pickles a little caffeine kick!

- A small amount (concentrations of up to 0.5 percent) of calcium chloride ("cackle") may be added to brine for cucumber pickles to act as an enzyme inhibitor. Calcium chloride is also used when curing olives. If you go this route, be sure to get food-grade calcium chloride, not the kind that you spread on sidewalks to melt ice!
- Aluminum sulfate ("alum") is also sometimes used in pickle making. It is a common ingredient in baking powder. Unfortunately, it is a neurotoxin and should be avoided.

Which Seasonings Should I Add?

Here are a few ideas about herbs, spices, and flavorings to get you started:

- Salt, probably. If you want to use less than a typical amount of salt, you may want to use more starter to ensure a good microbial balance.
- Dill is a classic seasoning for sour pickles; fennel and lovage suggest themselves as possibilities. Garlic and celery seed work well, too.
- A traditional "pickling spice" mix might contain red and black pepper, coriander, cumin, ginger, allspice, cinnamon, bay leaf, mustard seed, clove, and turmeric.
- Asian sauerkraut relatives, like kimchi, start with napa cabbage, daikon, or mustard greens; they often include ginger, garlic, onion, and hot red pepper; turmeric, galangal, and burdock are all welcome additions.
- South American sauerkrauts may include cabbage, red onion, carrot, oregano, and dried or fresh chile pepper; think about other members of the mint family, and/or cilantro. It's great to add olive oil when you're about to serve it.
- Carolina-style coleslaw, which was almost certainly fermented rather than vinegared a few generations ago, starts with cabbage, onion, green bell pepper, shredded carrot, mustard, and celery seed or root. Again, oil may be added when it's ready to be served.

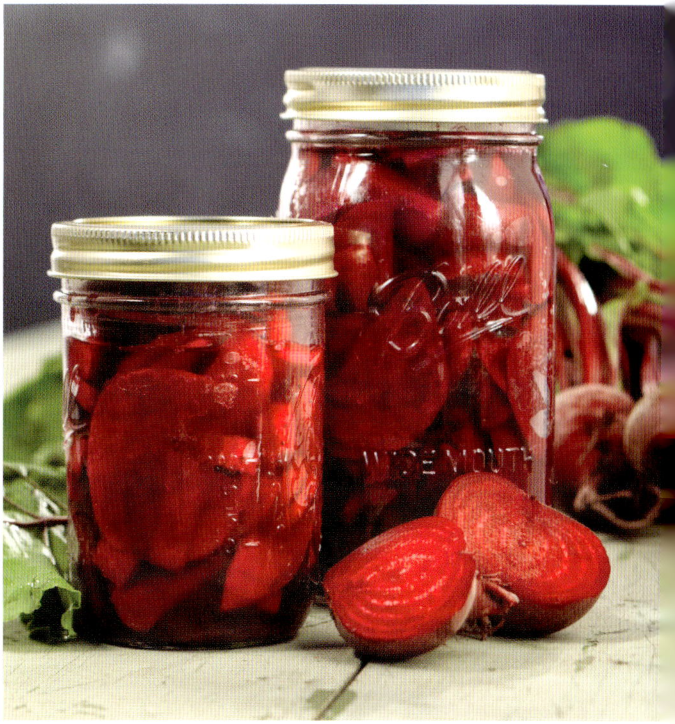

Lacto-Fermented Vegetables

PREP TIME: 10 MINUTES • TOTAL TIME: 4 DAYS–4 WEEKS

This recipe is very similar to the recipe for Basic Sauerkraut on page 39. Consider reading that one first for an in-depth introduction!

INGREDIENTS

2 pounds (1 kg) cabbage, turnips, radishes, kohlrabi, celery root, and/or other vegetables, as desired

4 teaspoons (20 g) sea salt

Seasonings, as desired

EQUIPMENT

Large cutting board (wood is ideal)

Large knife (a chef's knife is ideal)

Large mixing bowl

1-quart (1-L) mason jar, or similar glass jar with a tight-fitting lid

—

Yield: 1 quart (1 L)

PREPARATION

1. Peel, shred, core, seed, chop, and/or slice your vegetables, as desired. Carrots, turnips, beets, and the like may be peeled (a) (see page 43), and they may be shredded or cut (b).

2. Weigh all of the vegetables together, after you have peeled, cored, and otherwise prepped them.

3. Measure 2 teaspoons (10 g) of sea salt per pound (0.5 kg) of vegetables (or 2 percent salt by weight).

4. Combine the vegetables and the salt in the mixing bowl (c).

5. Massage them together forcefully with your hands, for a minute or two (d).

6. Pack the vegetables into the jar with your hands as tightly as possible (e).

7. Use a smaller jar, a bottle, a potato masher, some other rigid object, or simply your fingertips to pack the vegetables even more tightly into the jar. Ideally, when you push down, liquid will rise above the tops of the vegetables (f). Close the jar tightly.

8. Open the jar and pack its contents down a few times over the next couple of days with your fingertips.

Turnips and beets, cut into rounds or matchsticks, are a great combination (g). They get tender and juicy after several days. Add parsnips, too, cut into rounds, if you like (h).

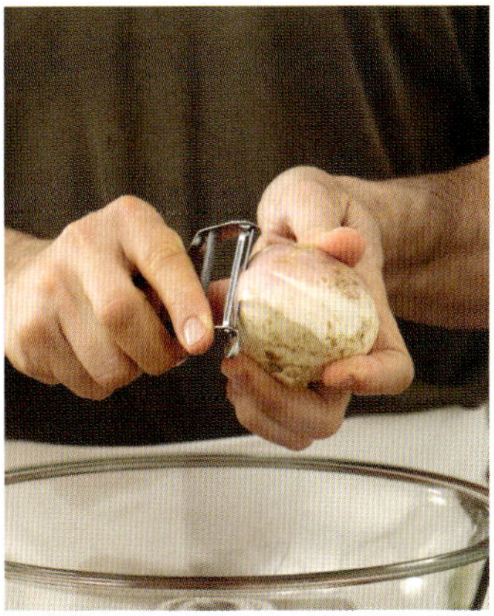

a

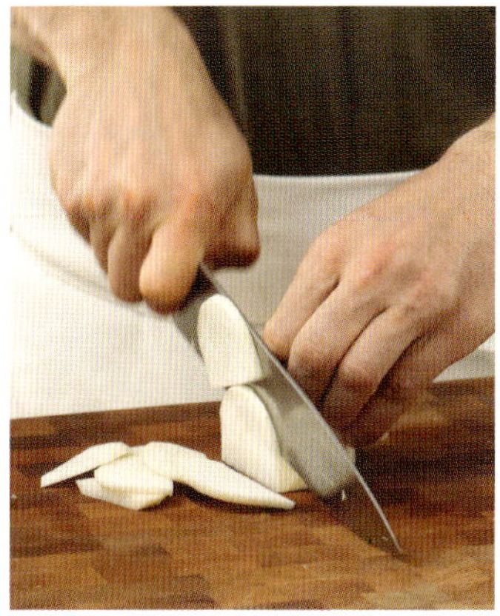

b

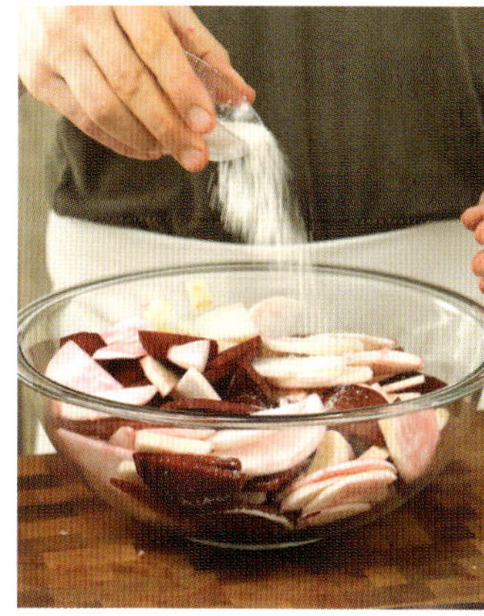

c

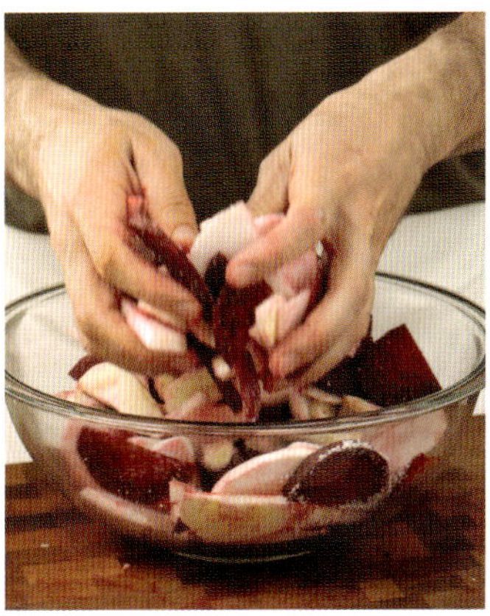

d

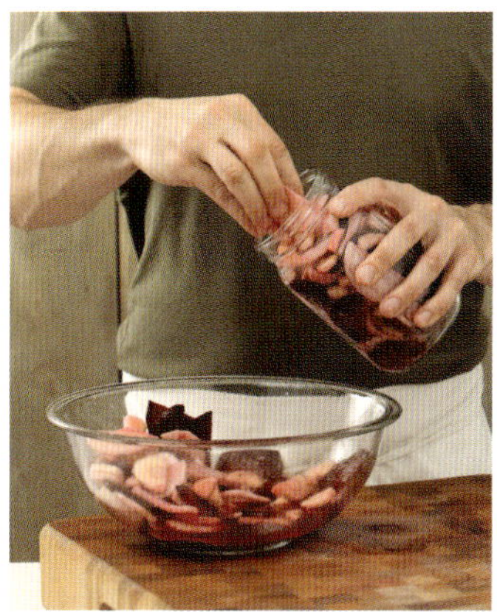

e

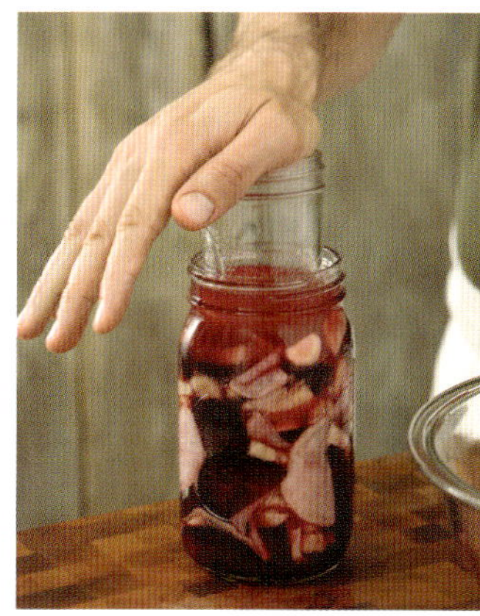

f

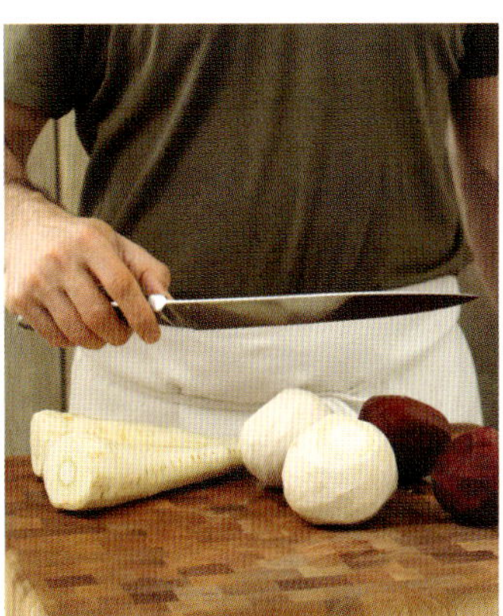

g

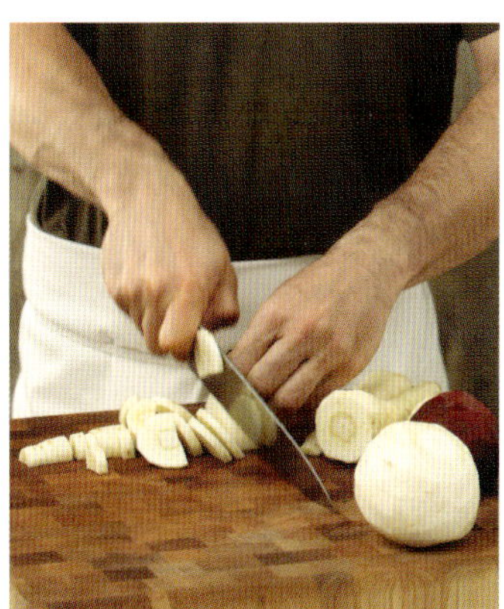

h

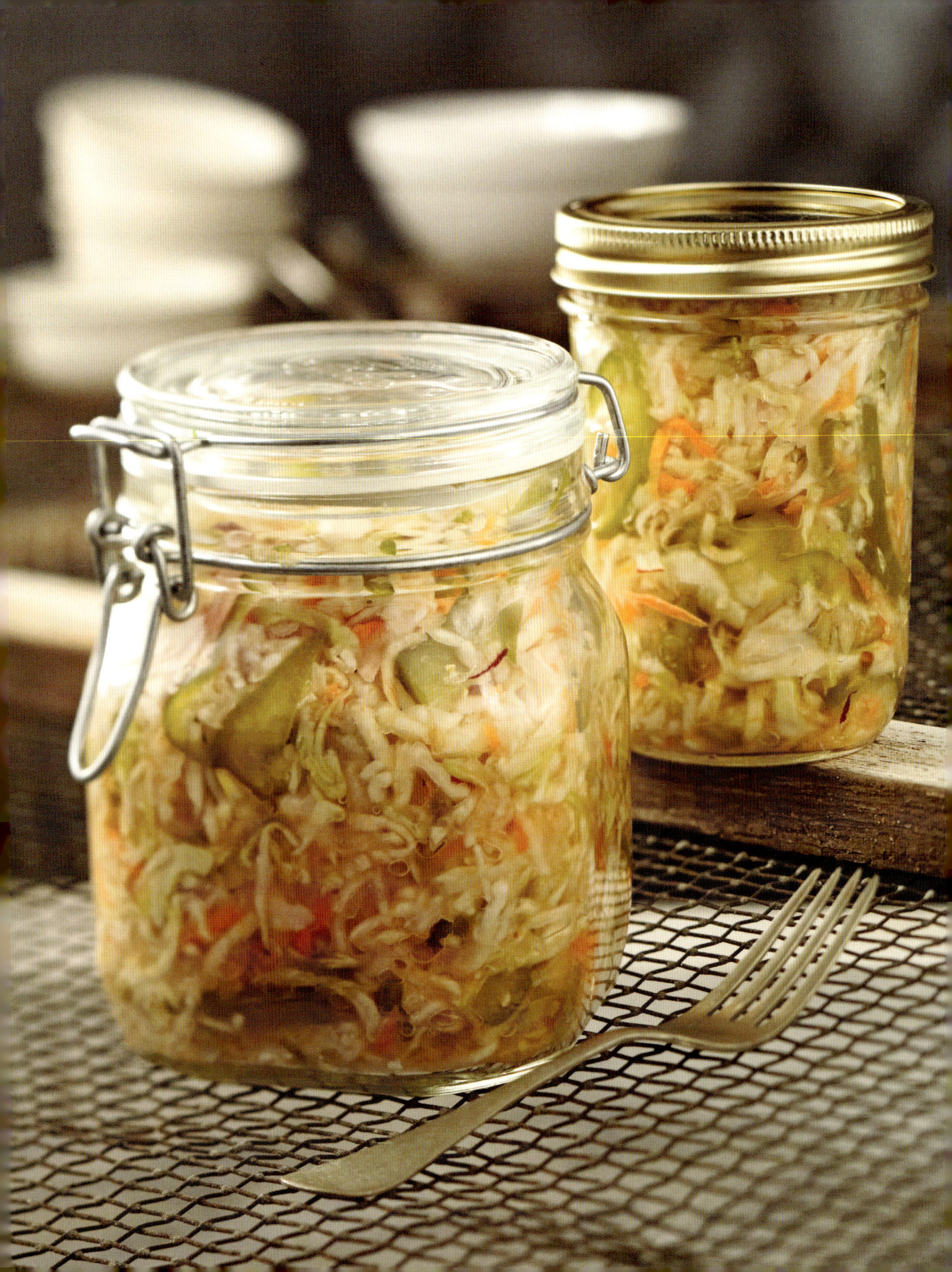

Fermented Carolina-Style Slaw

PREP TIME: 20 MINUTES • TOTAL TIME: 4–7 DAYS

Carolina-style slaw is a type of coleslaw that is traditional in the southeastern United States. The dressing for this coleslaw is similar to a vinaigrette salad dressing and does not contain mayonnaise or sour cream like some other sorts of coleslaw. I generally prefer Carolina-style coleslaw to the creamy kind. Especially if I'm having barbecued meats, for instance, or other heavy or fatty foods, a creamy slaw is "too much of the same"—I'm happier with a clean, crisp, and sour slaw.

It's clear to me that today's Carolina slaw, soured with vinegar, is a re-creation of the slaws of yesteryear, which must have been fermented—soured via bacterial action—because that was how one kept cabbage. I would like to bring back this fermented slaw. The big benefit, besides taste and texture, is that the fermentation process makes everything easier to digest—both the cabbage and whatever it's accompanying.

The same recipe can be made with whatever vegetables you like, selected according to the criteria outlined earlier in this chapter and in chapter 2. Cabbage relatives are good choices. Some possibilities include broccoli, cauliflower, Brussels sprouts, and shredded turnip. Or you could replace all the cabbage with celery root if you wanted to.

INGREDIENTS

1 pound (0.5 kg) green cabbage

1 large onion (red, yellow, or white)

1 large green bell pepper

1 large carrot

½ apple (optional)

¼ pound (115 g) celery root, or 1 teaspoon celery seed

4 teaspoons (20 g) sea salt

¼ cup (80 g) honey (or less, if you have included an apple)

6 tablespoons (90 ml) oil (a mixture of sesame, coconut, and olive oils works well)

2 teaspoons dry mustard

1 piece (⅓ inch, or 8 mm) gingerroot, peeled and grated (optional)

Freshly ground black pepper

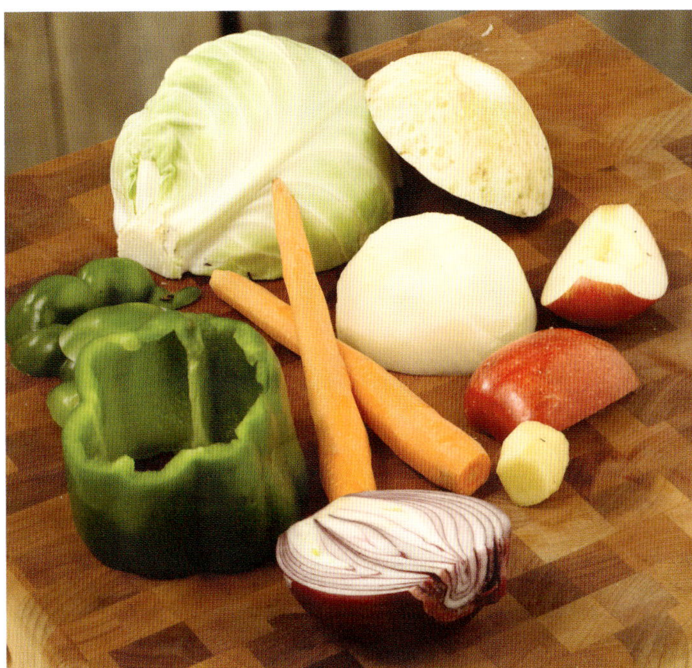

continued

Fermented Carolina-Style Slaw *(continued)*

EQUIPMENT
Large cutting board (wood is ideal)

Large knife (a chef's knife is ideal)

Large mixing bowl

2 mason jars (1 pint, or 500 ml each) or similar glass jars with tight-fitting lids

Colander or strainer

—

Yield: 1 quart (1 L), or 2 pounds (1 kg)

PREPARATION

1. Thinly slice the cabbage, onion, and bell pepper (a). (For tips on how to cut a bell pepper, see page 61.)

2. Grate or shred the carrot, apple, if using, and celery root, if using (b).

3. Ferment the vegetable mixture with the salt using the recipe for Lacto-Fermented Vegetables on page 46, to the desired degree of sourness (c), (d), (e). Four to seven days is probably about right.

4. Once the vegetables are fermented, drain them in a colander set over a mixing bowl, and press the liquid out with your hands, reserving the liquid.

5. Combine ½ cup (120 ml) of the liquid with the honey, oil, dry mustard, and ginger, and mix well with a fork, whisk, or blender (f), (g). Pour the dressing mixture into the mixing bowl (h), add the vegetables back in, and combine. Add salt and pepper as needed. Add more of the reserved liquid if you want more sourness. Refrigerate.

Save any leftover fermentation liquid to use as a starter for your next project. Or mix it with oil and spices to use as a salad dressing. Or drink it in the morning as a digestive tonic!

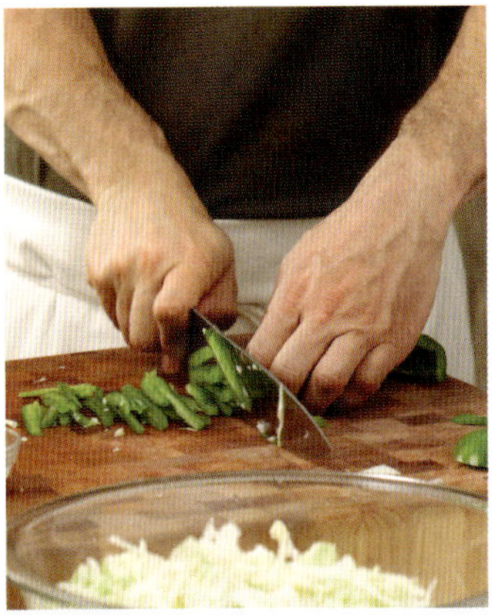

a

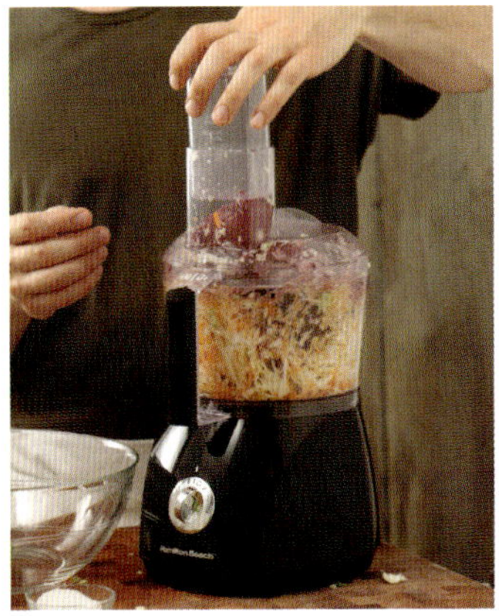

b

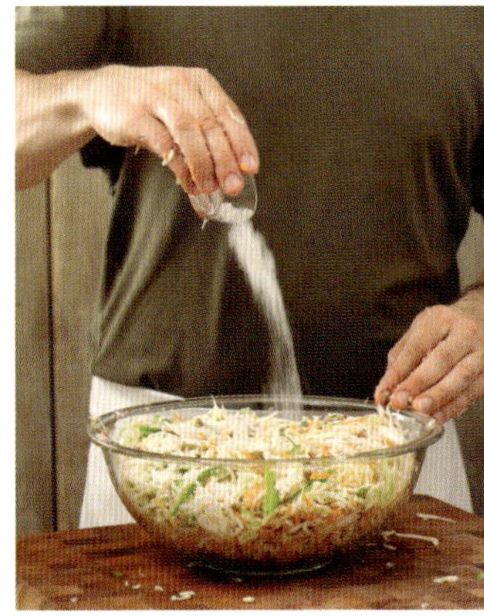

c

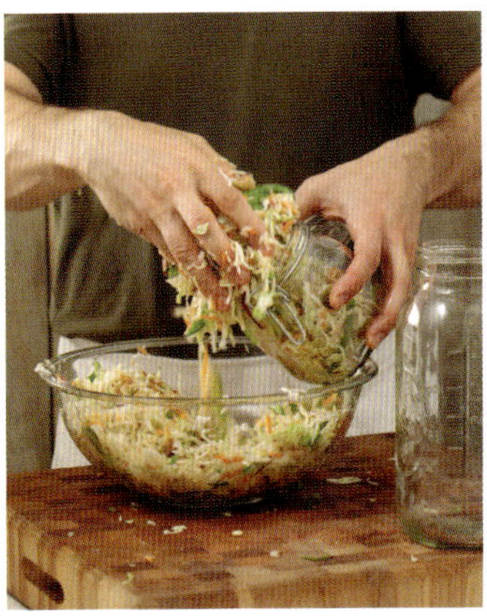

d

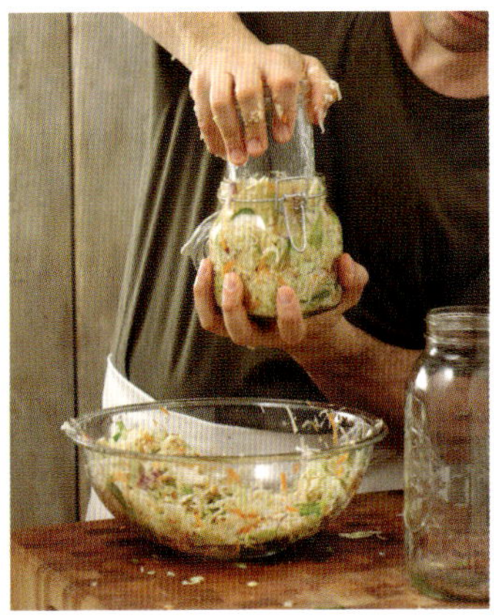

e

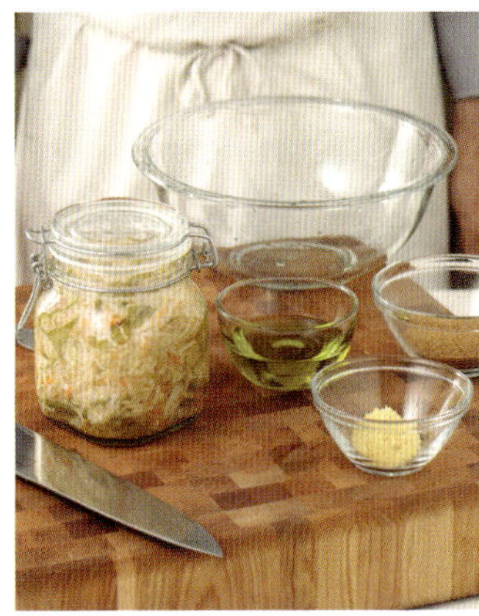

f

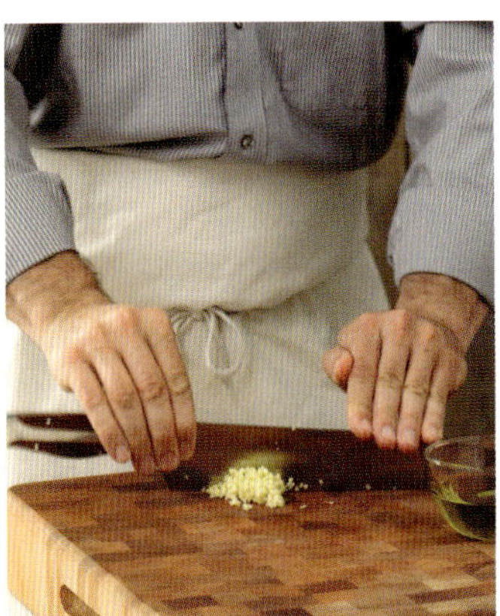

g

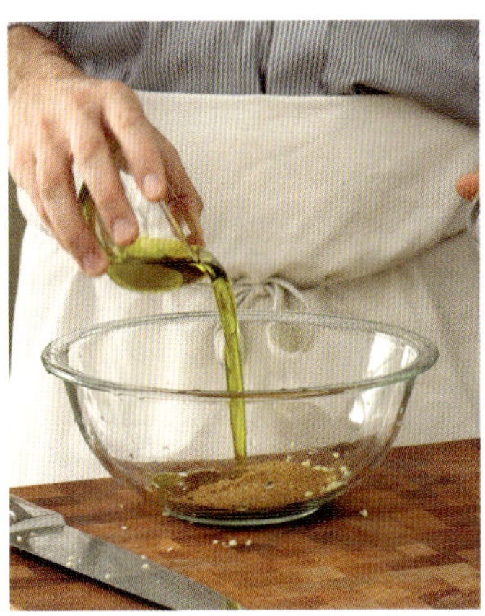

h

Cucumber Pickles

PREP TIME: 10 MINUTES • TOTAL TIME: 3 DAYS–2 WEEKS

Pickled cucumbers, or simply "pickles," are another quintessential fermented food. The first record of pickles comes from ancient Mesopotamia. Such diverse historical figures as Aristotle, Julius Caesar, Shakespeare, Amerigo Vespucci, and Thomas Jefferson are reported to have been fond of pickles. Indeed, Amerigo Vespucci, after whom America was named, was a pickle vendor before he became a world explorer.

Pickles play a significant role in the food culture of many countries, from North America through Europe and into the Middle East.

INGREDIENTS

About 3 pounds (1.5 kg) small, thick-skinned cucumbers, optionally cut in half or in quarters lengthwise

Chlorine-free water

3 tablespoons (40 g) sea salt

Seasonings: generous amounts of whole garlic, bay leaf, peppercorns, etc. (optional)

A few fresh grape or oak leaves, or a couple of black tea bags, for their tannins (optional)

Red wine vinegar or apple cider vinegar, boiled and cooled to replace some of the water (optional)

EQUIPMENT

Knife

Cutting board (wood is ideal)

½-gallon (2-L) mason or similar jar

—

Yield: About 3 pounds (1.5 kg)

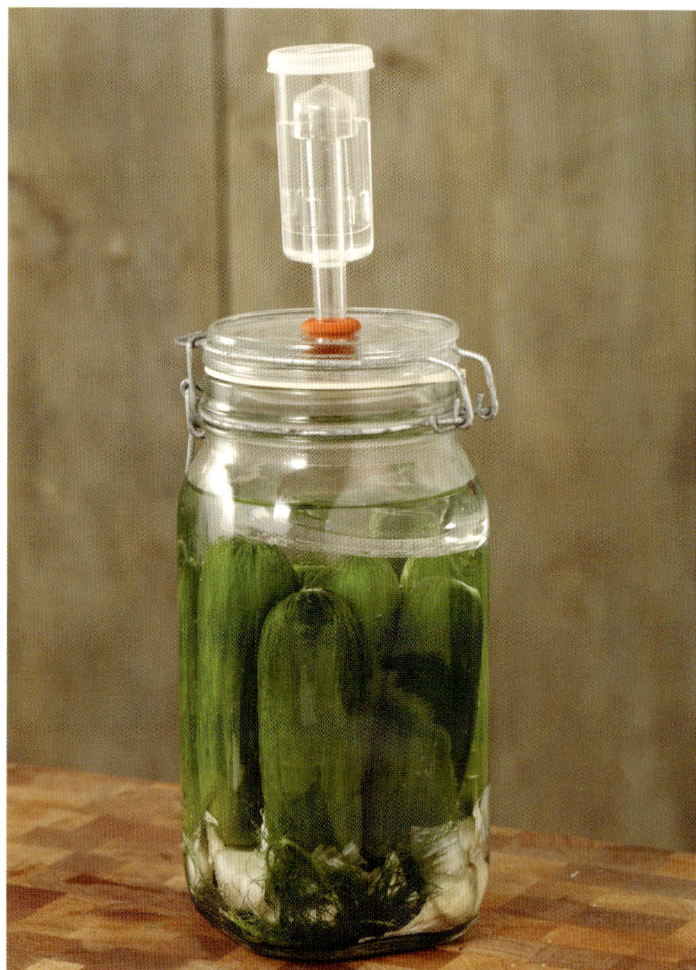

continued

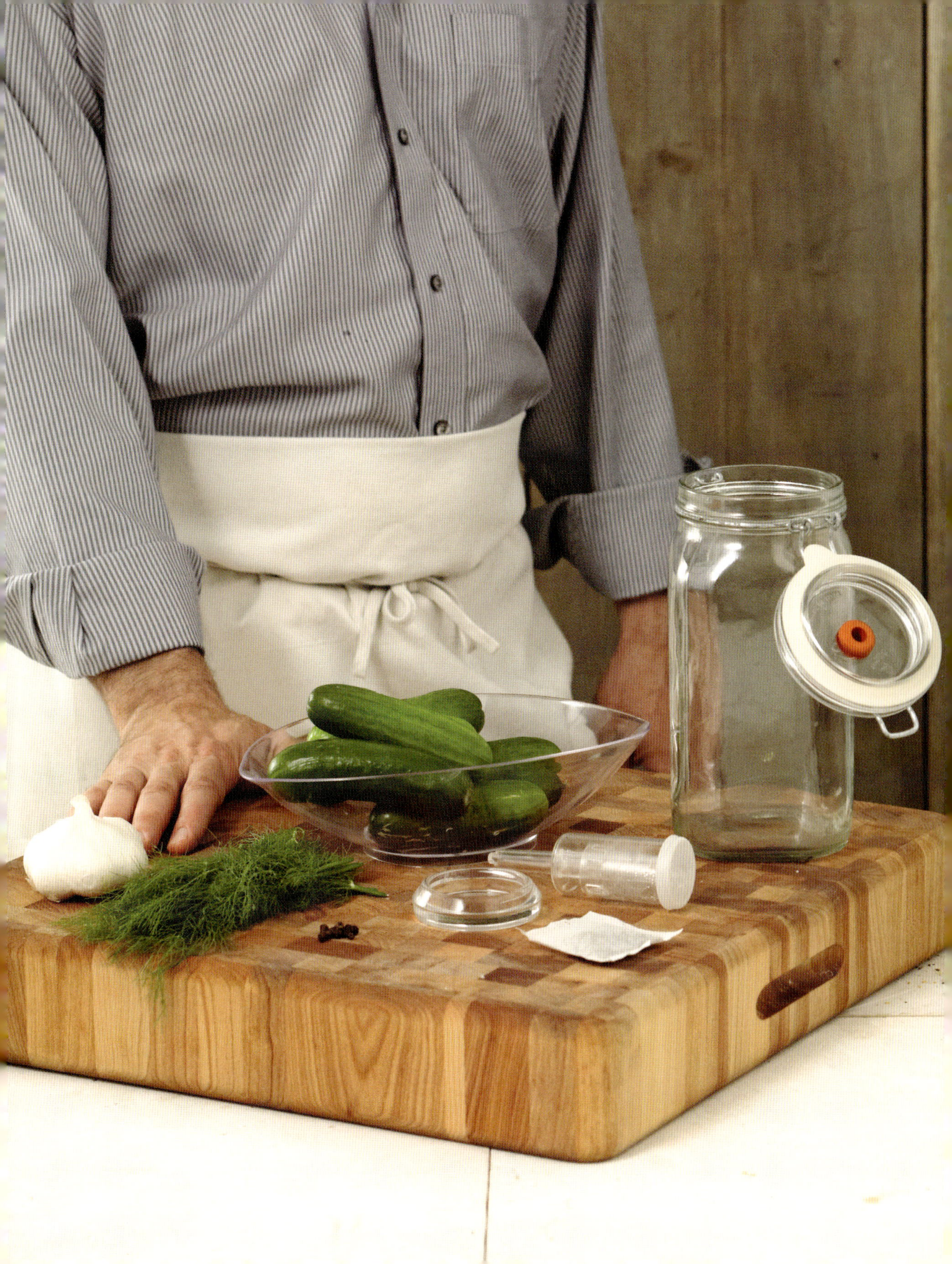

Cucumber Pickles *(continued)*

PREPARATION

1. If your cucumbers are at all soft, if you bought them at the store, and/or if you suspect that they might have been picked a while ago, you can perk them up by soaking them in ice water (a).

2. Trim the blossom ends off your cucumbers (b). These ends contain enzymes that can contribute to "hollow pickle syndrome" (see page 42).

3. Put the salt in the bottom of the mason jar. Add an inch or two of water. Swirl it until it is mostly dissolved.

4. Place the seasonings and tannin providers in the jar, followed by as many of the cucumbers as will fit (c).

5. Top off the container with water (d).

6. Weight everything down in such a way that it stays submerged (e) (optional).

7. Keep at cool room temperature, in a location where you won't forget about them. Every day after the second or third, pull out a pickle, cut off a piece with a clean knife, and taste it. When the pickles are pleasantly sour but still crunchy, they are done. Move them to a cool place (like the refrigerator) immediately.

If a little white stuff grows on the top of the brine, it's probably just yeast and it's not a problem—just remove it and carry on. But if there is a lot of white stuff, and it has long tendrils reaching down into the brine, it is a problem. Chalk one up to experience, send your pickles to the compost heap, and use more starter and/or vinegar next time.

See earlier in this chapter for pickle seasoning ideas and for suggestions about how to ensure the success of your pickles.

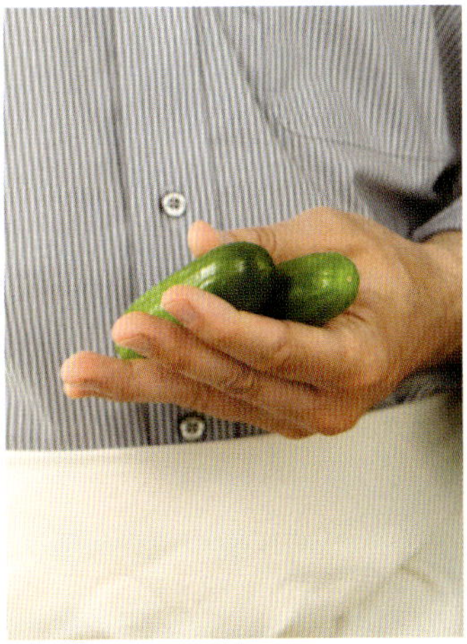

a

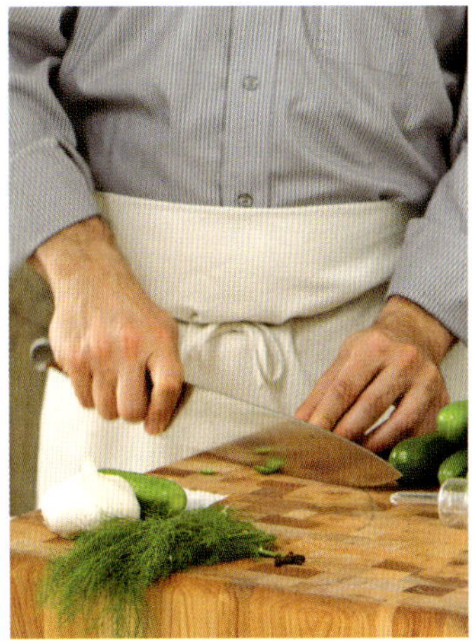

b

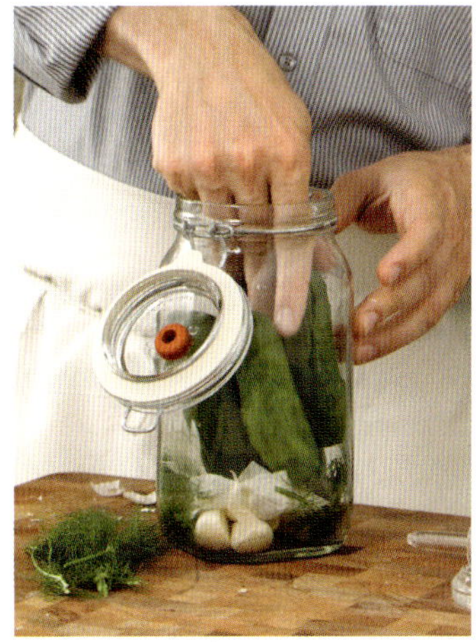

c

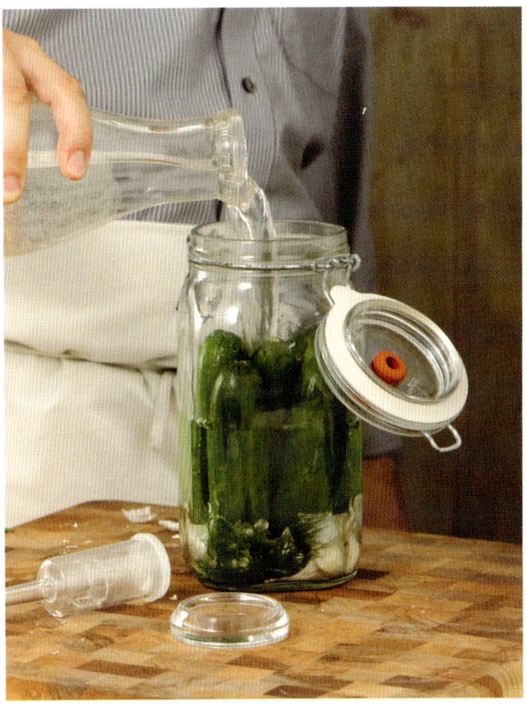

d

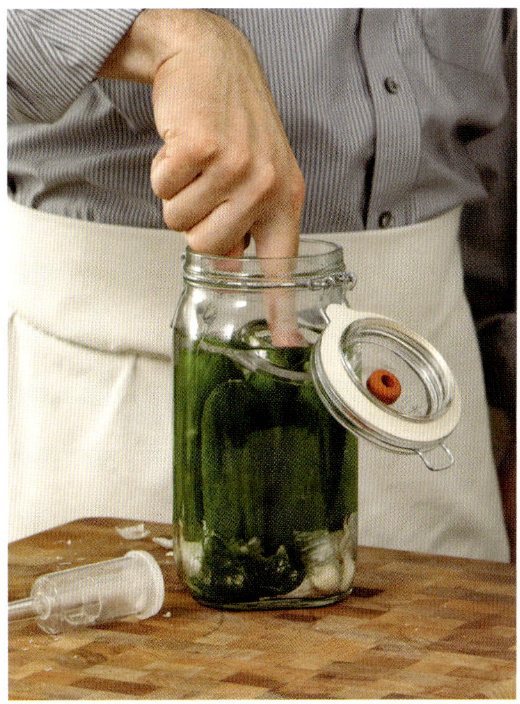

e

Kimchi

PREP TIME: 10 MINUTES + OVERNIGHT + 20 MINUTES • TOTAL TIME: 5 DAYS

Kimchi (also *gimchi* and, especially in Hawaii, *kimchee* or *kim chee*) is a Korean fermented vegetable dish. Kimchi can showcase a variety of vegetables, but kimchi made from napa cabbage, also known as celery cabbage or Chinese cabbage, is the most iconic.

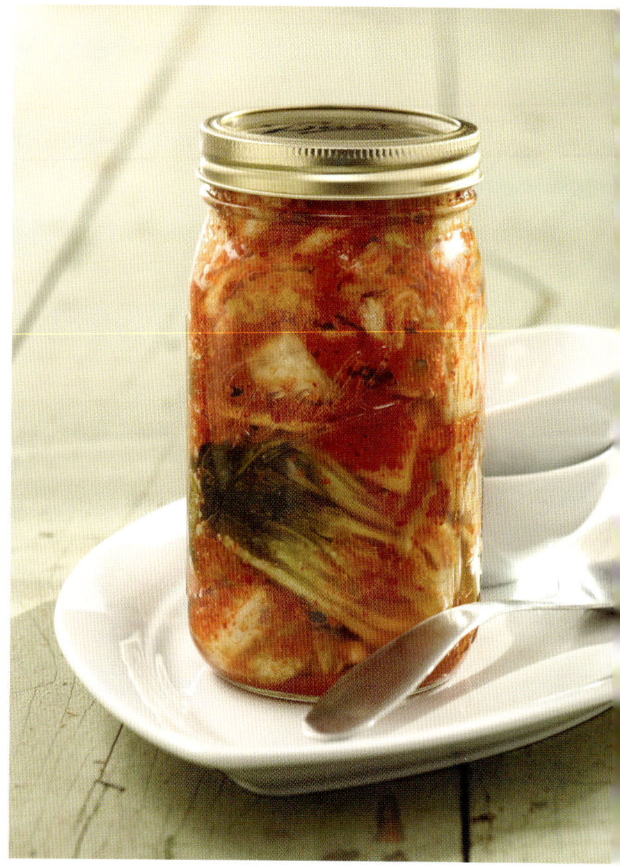

There's no one right or wrong way to spell "kimchi" in English (or to be more precise, in Roman characters). There is some amount of interpretation involved with transliterating words from one writing system into another, so it's possible to make a case for various spellings.

In my opinion, any fermented vegetable mix containing cruciferous vegetables (such as cabbage or radish), allium (such as garlic, onion, or scallion), ginger, and salt may safely be called kimchi. Other combinations of ingredients are also sometimes called kimchi.

Red pepper features prominently in many kimchis, but not in all of them. In fact, the first historical record of preserved cabbage in Asia predates the introduction of red pepper, a New World spice, by at least 2,000 years; so in relative terms, red pepper is a recent addition to kimchi.

Some might say that kimchi is a Korean sort of sauerkraut; others would say that sauerkraut is a European version of kimchi. In fact, the oldest known preserved cabbage was in China, so it may in fact be the Chinese who have the best claim to primacy.

INGREDIENTS

⅓ cup (100 g) coarse salt

2 cups (500 ml) nonchlorinated water

2 pounds (1 kg) vegetables: napa cabbage, plus optional mustard greens, bok choy, or daikon

½ head garlic

1 large or 2 small onions

1 piece (½ inch, or 13 mm) gingerroot

Up to ½ cup (30 g) Korean red pepper powder, chopped or ground red peppers, or pepper flakes

1 tablespoon (15 g) sugar

1 teaspoon or more fish sauce (optional)

a few scallions or a length of Korean "long onion" (which is, more or less, a mature scallion)

EQUIPMENT

Large mixing bowl

Large knife (a chef's knife is ideal)

Large cutting board (wood is ideal)

Vegetable peeler

Colander

Food processor (optional)

continued

PREPARATION

1. In the mixing bowl, dissolve the salt in the water to make a brine.

2. Cut up any or all of the 2 pounds (1 kg) of vegetables: Quarter the leafy bunches of vegetables, or cut them into 1-inch (2.5 cm) square pieces. Slice the cabbage core and include as much or as little as you like. Peel the root vegetables, and cut them into thin diagonal slices, 1 inch (2.5 cm) or so long.

3. Put the cut vegetables into the brine and mix, using clean hands. The brine makes the vegetables more malleable. Cover the bowl to keep it free of foreign objects. After 6 or so hours (or overnight), drain the vegetables thoroughly in a colander. Taste them. They should be salty, but not unpleasantly so. If they are unpleasantly salty, rinse them or soak them in fresh nonchlorinated water, taste them again, and repeat until you are satisfied. Set them aside.

4. Peel the garlic and the onions. Peel the ginger (the edge of a spoon works nicely) (a).

5. Blend the onions, garlic, and ginger in a food processor (b), adding enough water to allow them to blend (c). (Or mix them with a mortar and pestle, or chop them finely with a knife.)

6. Add the red pepper (d), sugar, and fish sauce, if using, to the combination from step 5, adding just enough water to keep things blending into a paste.

7. Cut the scallions diagonally into 1-inch (2.5-cm) lengths (e), add them to the paste, and mix the paste with a wooden spoon.

continued

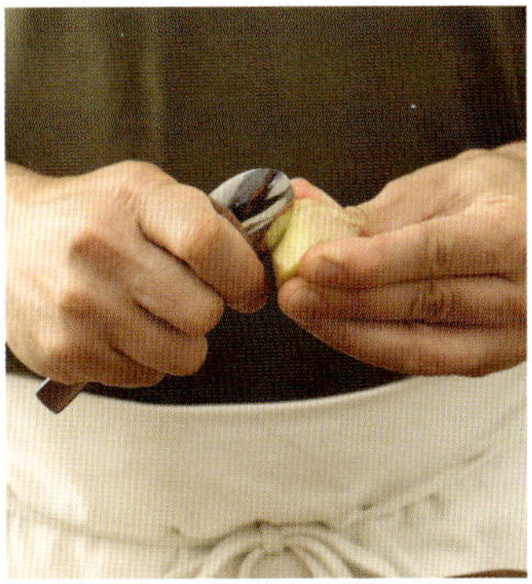

a

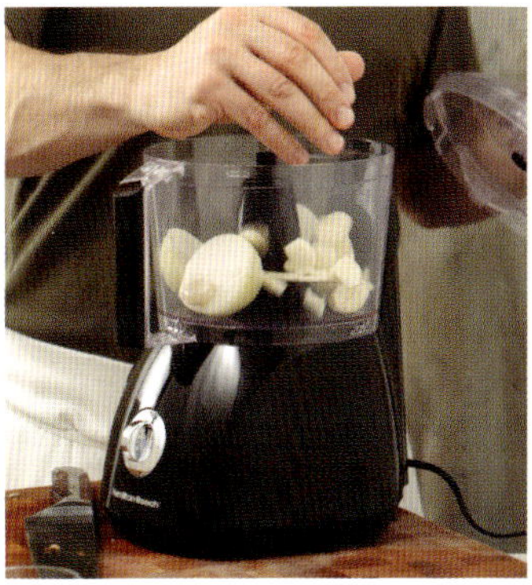

b

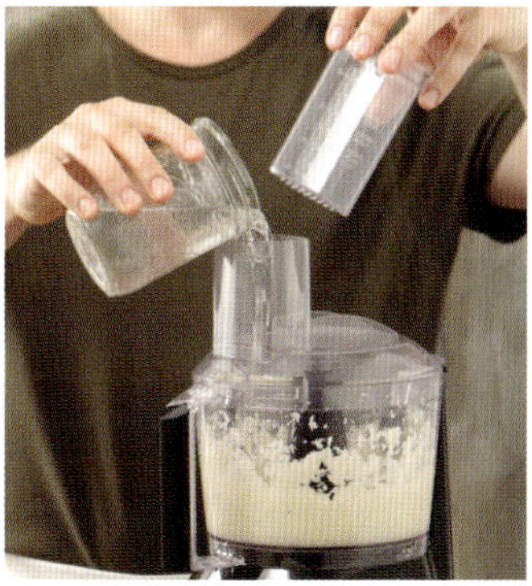

c

Kimchi *(continued)*

Wooden spoon

Wide-mouthed mason jars (2 pints [500 ml each], or 1 quart [1 L])

—

Yield: Approximately 1 quart (1 L), or 2 pounds (1 kg)

8. Move the drained vegetables into a large bowl (f), and mix them with the seasoning paste using the spoon (g), (h). Taste the kimchi. If it is not salty enough, add more salt or fish sauce now and stir.

9. Pack the kimchi tightly into the Mason jars, leaving 1 inch (2.5 cm) of space at the top. Try to pack it down well enough to squeeze out most of the air bubbles along the side of the jar (i). Close the jar.

10. Leave the jar on the counter at room temperature for a few days. Taste it every day or two. It should start to taste a bit "wild." When you like the way it tastes, put it in a cool cellar or a refrigerator to store, or bury it in the ground. The cooler the temperature, the slower the subsequent fermentation.

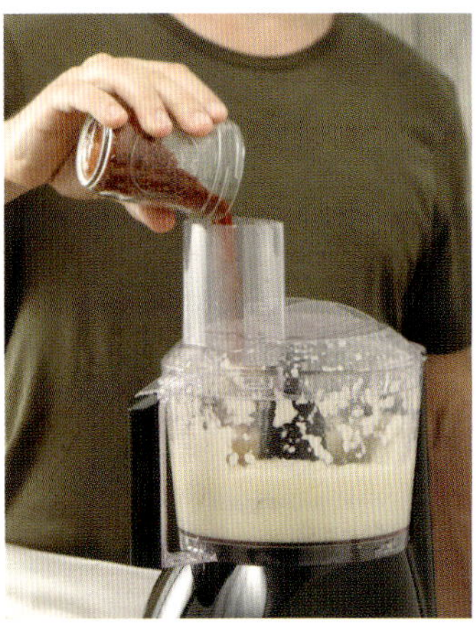

d

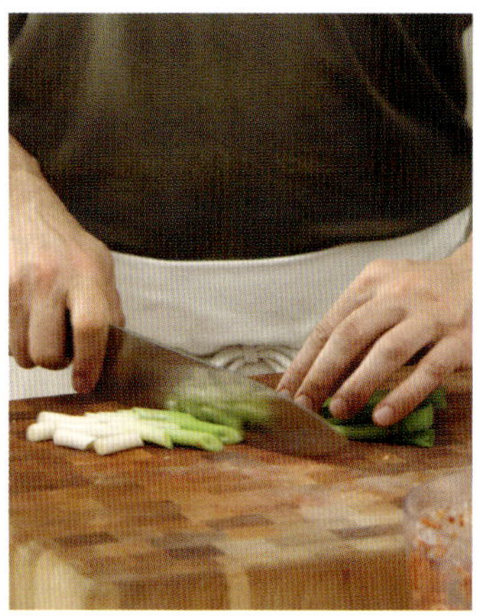

e

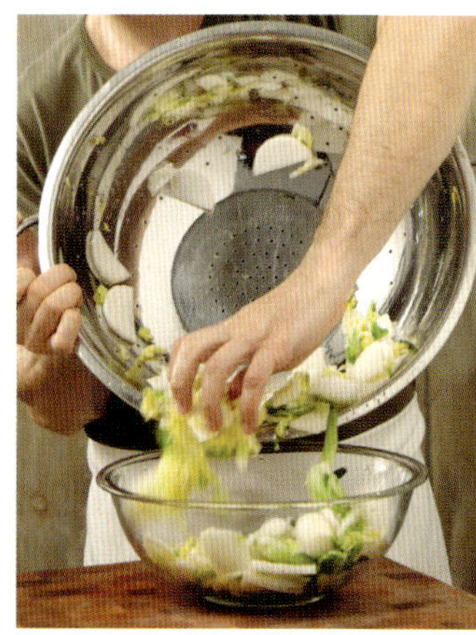

f

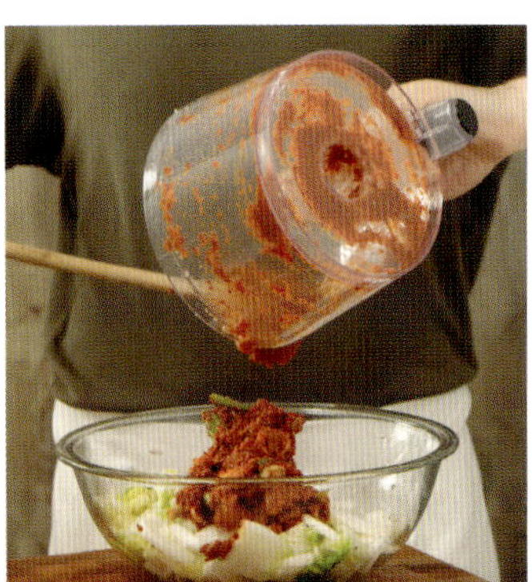

g

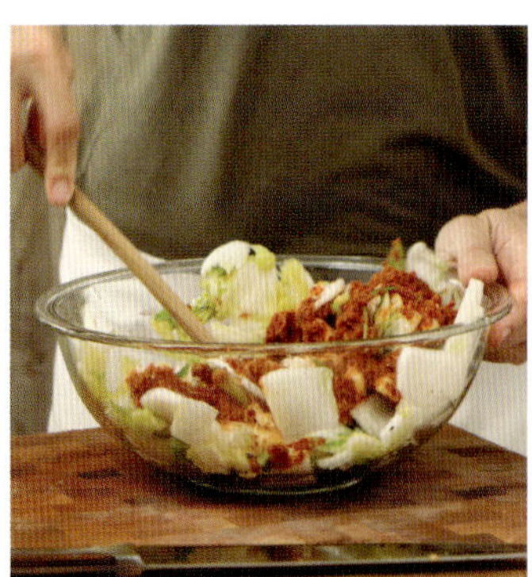

h

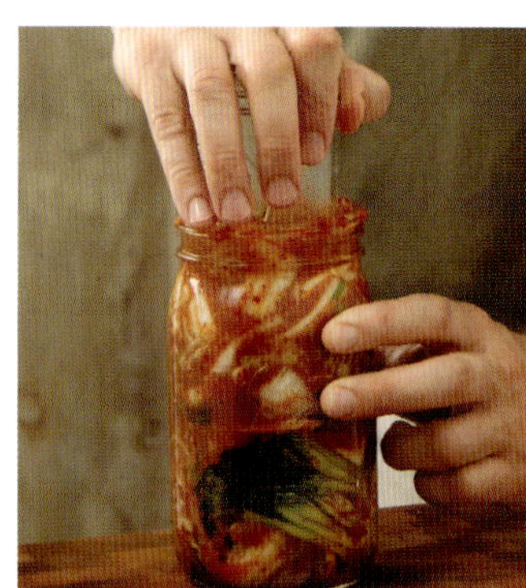

i

CUTTING NAPA CABBAGE AND DAIKON

Napa cabbages (a) are typically more cylindrical than other varieties of cabbage, which are more spherical.

This makes napa cabbage easy to work with. Once you cut it in half the long way (b), (c), you can lay it down on your cutting board and quarter it (d), then start cutting it into even widths (e).

Daikon is equally convenient to handle. Rather than being small and round, it is large and cylindrical. So you can cut it lengthwise (f), and then easily slice it (g).

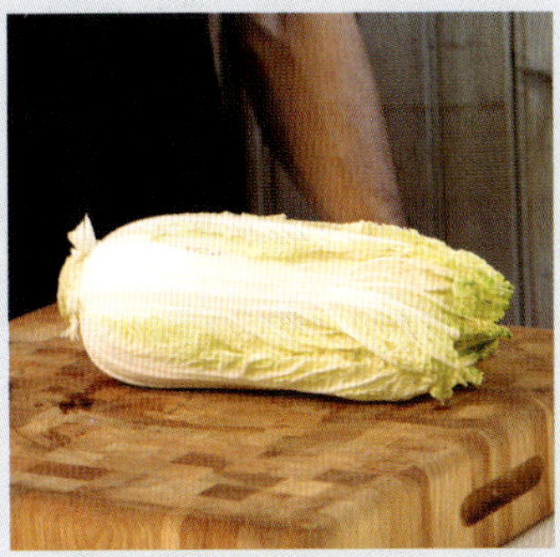

a

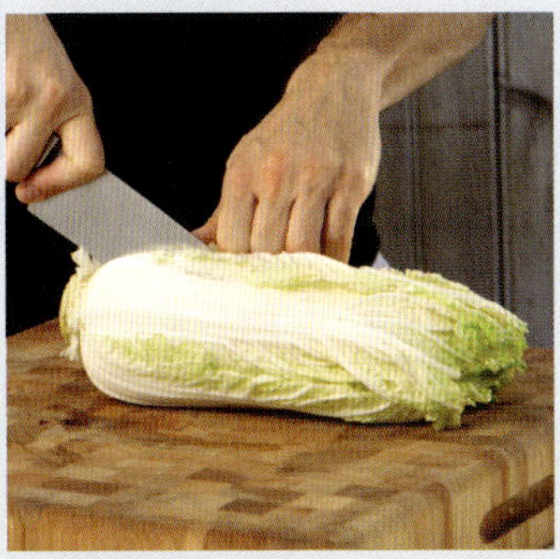

b

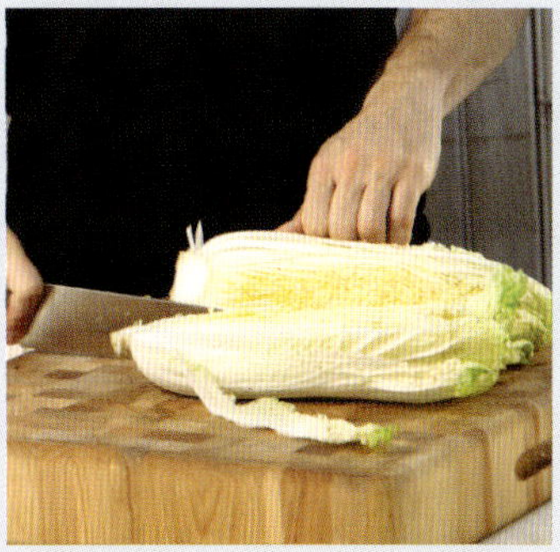

c

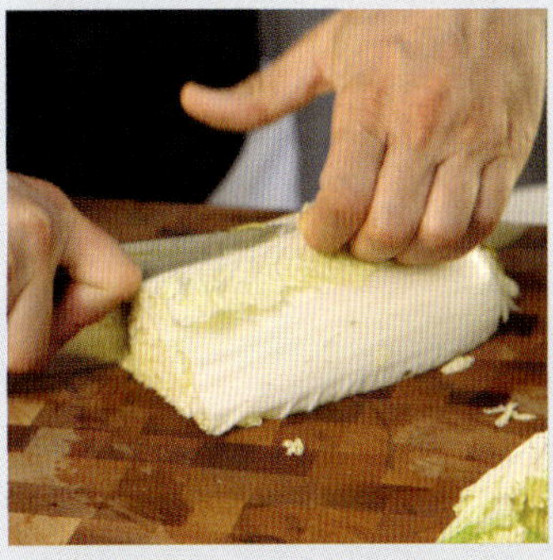

d

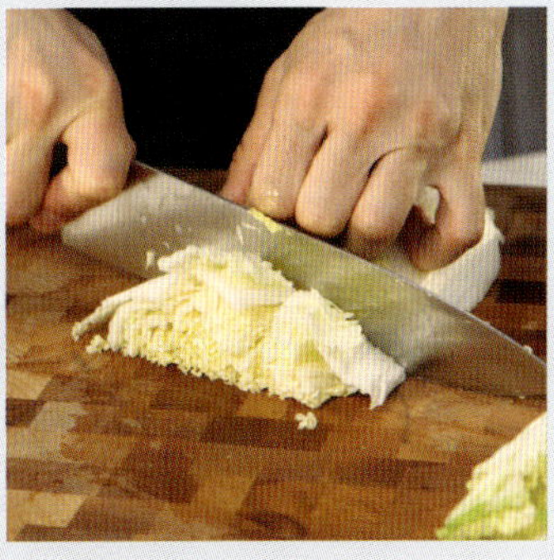

e

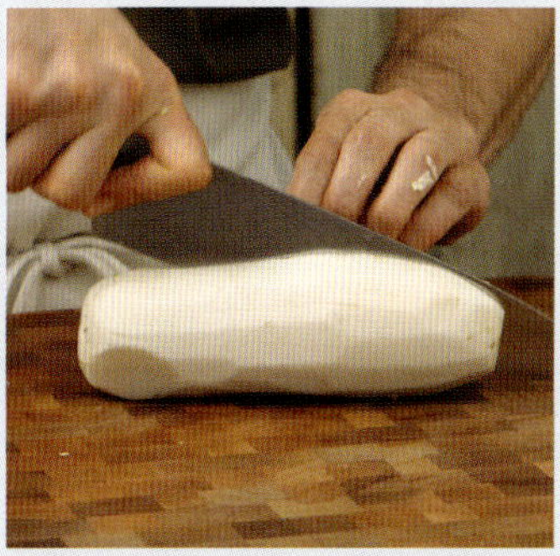

f

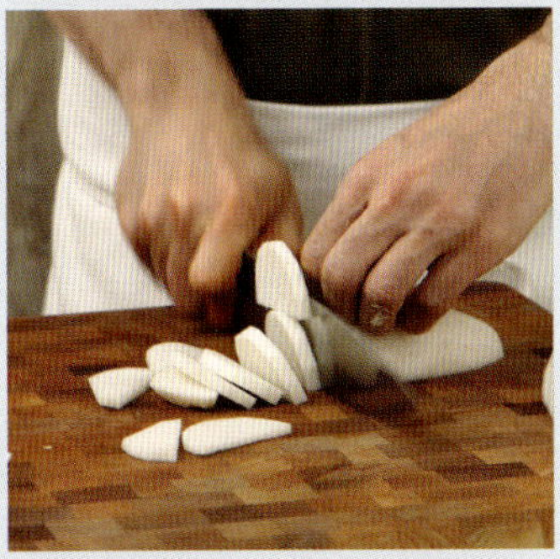

g

Serving Ideas for Kimchi

- Fresh kimchi is great with grilled or smoked foods and goes especially nicely with pork and/or apples. So grilled pork chops, pulled pork, and grilled mackerel or seared tuna would go nicely with kimchi.
- Kimchi can take the place of plain sauerkraut in many contexts. For instance, if you use kimchi instead of sauerkraut, a Reuben sandwich becomes a Kimchi Reuben sandwich, adding a whole new dimension to the classic. (By the way, corned beef is often fermented.)
- Older, less crunchy kimchi can be used in cooked preparations like soups and stews, egg dishes, savory pancakes, and fried rice. *Kimchi jjigae* is a kimchi stew popular in Korea. Kimchi scrambled eggs might be just the thing on a cold winter morning.
- You can make a kimchi canapé with a cracker, an oatcake, or a toast square topped with Cheddar cheese, a slice of crispy apple, and a dollop of finely chopped kimchi. Raise some eyebrows at your next cocktail party!
- Grilled cheese with kimchi is another nice variation on a comfort food favorite.
- Top your baked potato with sour cream and kimchi. (Sour cream, as you might guess, is fermented, too; see page 79.)
- Try oysters on the half shell with kimchi juice. Who needs hot sauce and lemon?
- Kimchi nachos provide a new and tasty flavor.
- Kimchitini! Have a vodka cocktail with a hint of kimchi juice . . . or a big splash if you like it dirty.
- A kimchi Bloody Mary is perfect with brunch.
- For a Kimchi Michelada, combine a light-bodied beer, kimchi juice, and lime juice over ice in a salt-rimmed glass. It's cold and refreshing on a hot summer day.

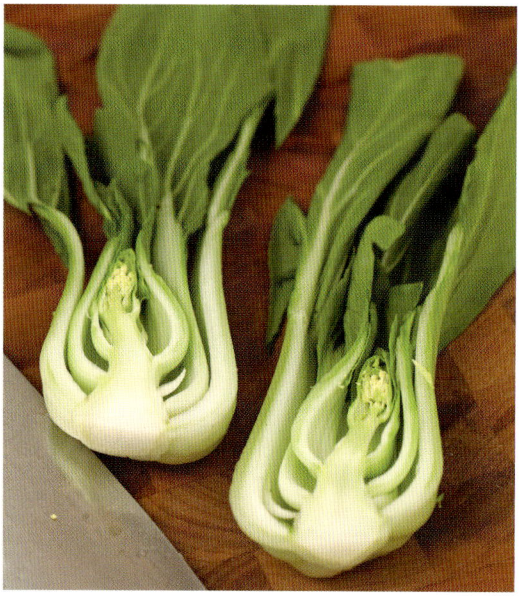

CUTTING A BELL PEPPER

This is a great process for cutting a bell pepper. It's particularly useful when readying bell peppers for fermentation, as in the recipe on page 49 for Fermented Carolina-Style Slaw.

1. Cut both top and bottom off the pepper (a), (b).

2. Run your knife around the inside of the pepper (c).

3. Put down your knife, and eject the seeds and core of the pepper by pushing with your thumbs (d).

4. Cut the pepper vertically (e) and lay it flat (f), or cut it into rings, or cut it however you want. Use the end pieces, too, if you like.

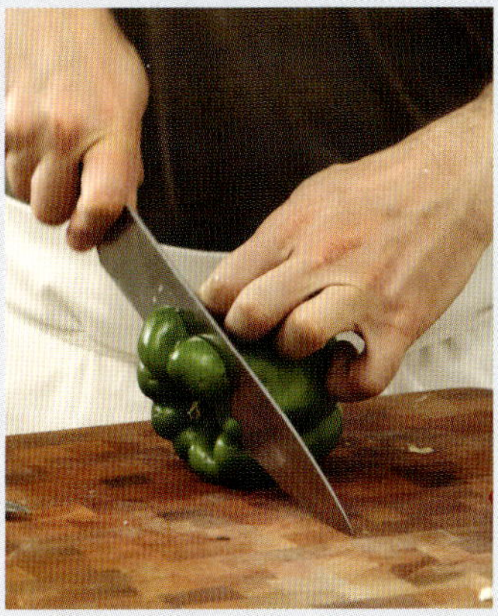

a

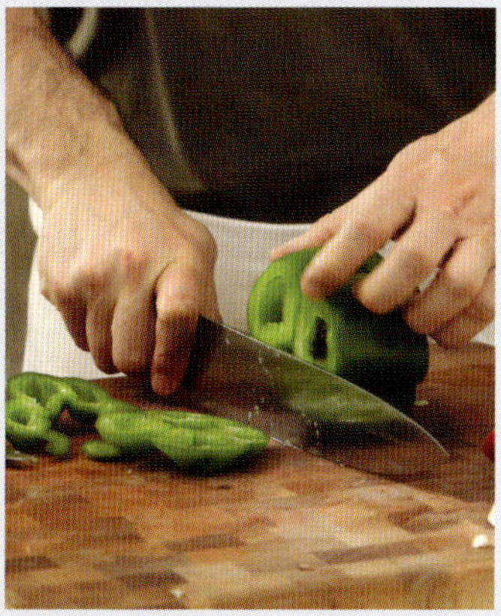

b

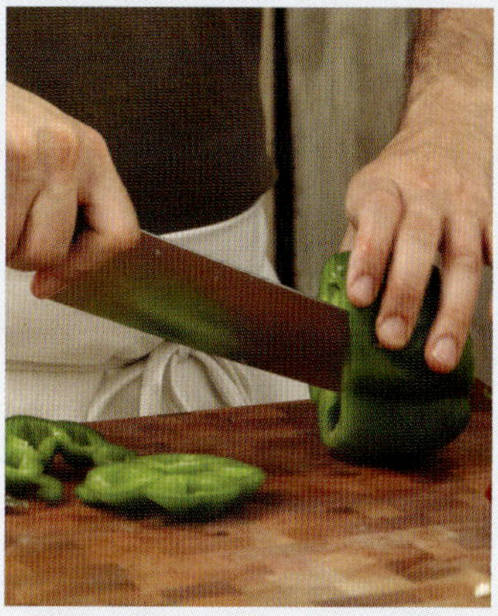

c

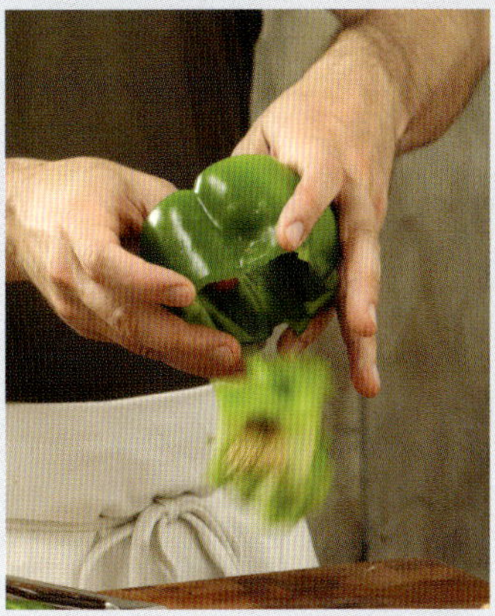

d

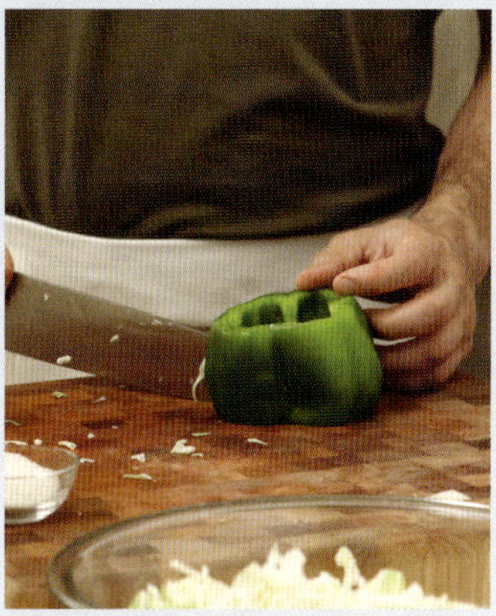

e

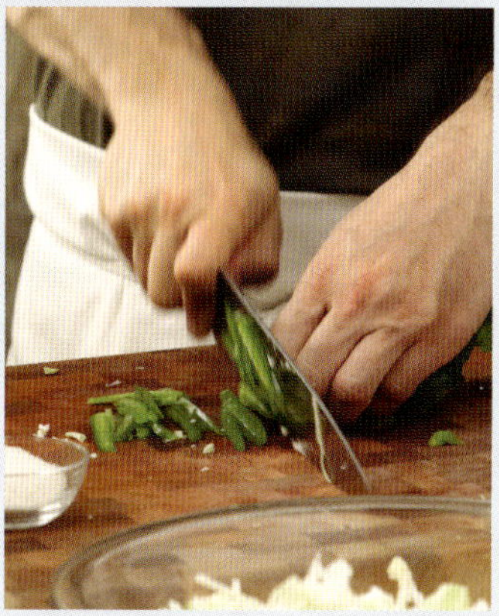

f

Nattō

PREP TIME: 20 MINUTES • TOTAL TIME: 28 HOURS

Natto (*nattō*) is a ferment from Japan made by introducing a specific bacterial culture, Bacillus subtilis var. natto, to warm cooked soybeans. Historically, natto was made by wrapping cooked soybeans in straw, which naturally hosts the desired bacteria. Today, natto is more often made from isolated spores (*nattomoto*). If you have a Japanese goods store near you, they may sell these spores in small envelopes; otherwise, look on the Internet. My most recent envelope of spores is Kawashima brand, purchased from thejapanstore.jp by way of Amazon.com. A 3-gram envelope is sufficient for at least 30 pounds (15 kg) of cooked soybeans, which translates to over 250 generous (2-ounce [60-g]) servings of natto.

I was introduced to natto by a friend and mentor, Steve-san. One day I was sitting with him before dinner at his amazing restaurant, Sawa Sushi, in Sunnyvale, California. He was eating some natto. I had read about natto and had not yet made up my mind to try it, so I asked him about it. Before I knew it, Steve had disappeared into the kitchen. He reappeared bearing a bowl of rice topped with a generous portion of natto. I couldn't very well refuse it at that point!

Natto is famous for its texture, called neba-neba in Japanese. In English, we might say "mucilaginous" or maybe "slippery" or "slimy." Okra and Japanese mountain yam (*naga-imo*) are two other neba-neba foods.

My first time eating natto was memorable. I had been warned about the texture, but it was surprising nonetheless—even before it reached my mouth. The natto soybeans I picked up trailed strands of neba-neba back to their companions in the bowl. It was a little like trying to pick up very thin noodles, twirling my chopsticks ineffectively.

Natto is soft in the mouth, having been thoroughly cooked and then fermented. It has a distinctive smell and flavor, a bit like a very ripe cheese, or perhaps ammonia-like, depending on whom you ask.

A NOTE ABOUT EQUIPMENT

In order to get consistent results making natto, you need to do two things: (1) cook soybeans, and (2) incubate them at 104°F (40°C) for 24 hours or so. It sounds simple enough!

The current generation of electric pressure cookers can do both of these things very well, so I use one and I recommend it. If you don't have one, you can cook the soybeans in whatever way you typically cook beans—a normal saucepan or stockpot will do. Then you will need to find a way to incubate with good temperature control. Some yogurt makers will be able to do this. I don't recommend using the oven to incubate, both because it will prevent anyone else from using the oven for 24 hours and also because most ovens don't have good temperature control in that range if they have any at all.

A NOTE ABOUT PROCESS

Natto (like many protein ferments) is more finicky than typical vegetable ferments.

Be as tidy as you can with your containers and tools and as sterile as is feasible in a home kitchen. The natto is most vulnerable from when the soybeans are cooked until the inoculated soybeans are safely incubating. Any utensils or tools you use during this window of time should be sterilized. Pouring boiling water over the utensils and tools is a reasonable way to do this.

The soybeans should be incubated in a layer a few beans thick in a shallow container, with some access to air, but not so much that they will dry out. If you are using the electric pressure cooker, this recipe will guide you easily; but if not, you may have to improvise based on the equipment you are using.

I enjoyed my natto that day with its typical garnishes of a little mustard, sweet soy sauce, and long onion (similar to scallion). It left me satisfied. I didn't crave more immediately, but once I had integrated the experience of eating it, I found myself wanting to try it again. And I have had it many times since.

Whether or not you are a fan, there is no denying that natto is exceptionally nutritious. I generally avoid using the term superfood because I think it's thrown around way too casually, but if it applies to anything, it applies to natto.

Natto contains nattokinase and vitamin K2 MK-7, substances that are unavailable (nattokinase) or much less available (K2 MK-7) from any other food. In scientific studies, nattokinase has mitigated blood clots and has demonstrated various additional salutary effects; K2 helps with bone density, heart health, and other things. Natto also contains more of the "usual" vitamins than unfermented soy, which is typical for a fermented food, since vitamins are common byproducts of microbe fermentation metabolism.

Soybeans are rich in minerals to start with, but unfermented soy contains large amounts of phytic acid, which blocks the absorption of calcium, magnesium, and zinc. Fermentation neutralizes the phytic acid, making the minerals in natto more bioavailable than in tofu or soy milk, for example.

Natto is also an exceptional source of soluble fiber. This fiber is evidenced by natto's neba-neba texture. The scientific consensus is that soluble fiber is good for digestion and for serum cholesterol regulation.

continued

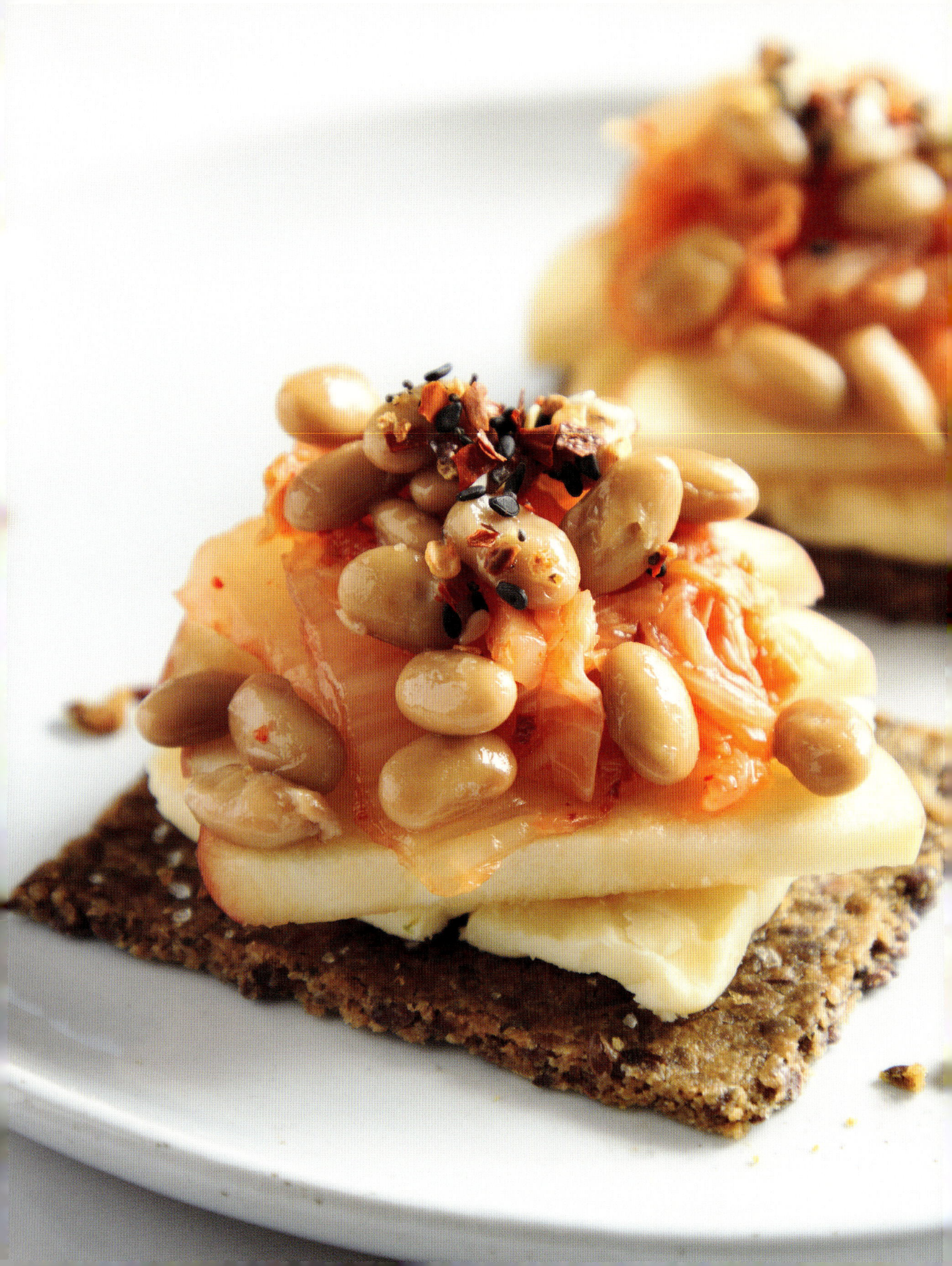

Natto *(continued)*

If you haven't had natto before, I would recommend buying some ready-to-eat natto and trying it before you dive into making it. Otherwise, you won't know how it could taste, and you won't know whether or not you love it! Ready-to-eat natto is available in the freezer section at most Japanese grocery stores and at some other Asian grocery stores. You can also find it on the Internet, of course. Some excellent small-volume natto producers are starting to pop up outside Japan. Try a few of these and try some of the Japanese exports and see which you like best!

This recipe makes a small batch of natto. Starting with small batches will allow you to perfect your process and develop your taste without filling your entire fridge and freezer with natto. You can scale up the recipe, but be aware that the inoculated soybeans need to be spread out thinly while fermenting so that they can have access to air. If you want to make a lot more natto than in this recipe, you may need to come up with a different incubation plan.

Most natto recipes talk about placing a porous layer of plastic wrap or parchment or equivalent on top of the natto for incubation. I've tried it with and without, and I have not noticed a difference. I suspect the controlled climate of my incubator is a factor. Regardless, in the spirit of simplicity, my recipe does not use a layer of wrap on top of the natto.

INGREDIENTS

1 cup (180 g) dry soybeans (small soybeans if you have a choice)

½ tiny spoon of natto spores (nattomoto, usually packaged in an envelope), using the tiny spoon that is included with the spores, or as directed in the spore instructions

Water sufficient to cook the soybeans, plus a cup or two more for sterilizing and for mixing with spores

—

2–3 cups natto

EQUIPMENT

Electric pressure cooker/proofer, or a way to cook soybeans and a way to incubate them

Strainer (possibly one that fits inside your cooker)

Small, airtight containers sufficient to store your natto (4-ounce [120-ml] containers are ideal, but anything smallish is okay)

PREPARATION

1. Cook your soybeans until tender and soft but not split. If you are using an electric pressure cooker, follow the manufacturer's instructions regarding cooking time, and use a time at the upper end of the recommended range.

(If you have a strainer that fits inside your cooking vessel, you can cook the soybeans in the strainer, which makes it easier to strain them in the next step.)

2. Strain. If you have cooked the beans inside a strainer, then pull the strainer out, dump the water from the cooker, and dump the strained beans back into the cooker. If you're doing it another way,

continued

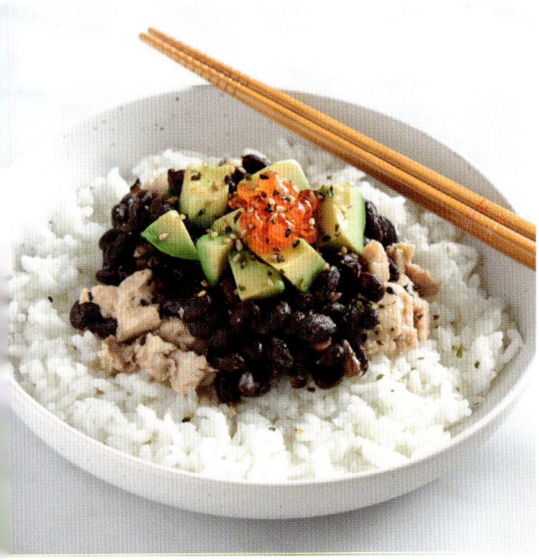

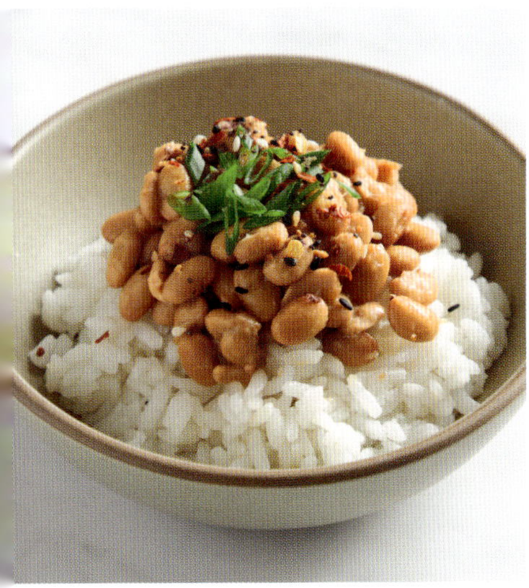

Natto *(continued)*

then remember to sterilize any tools that you use and make sure that the soybeans wind up in a thin layer, a few beans deep, in the vessel or vessels that you will use for incubation.

You can let the soybeans cool while you move on to the next step.

3. Boil some water and use that water to sterilize a large metal spoon, a small dish or bowl, or even a metal quarter-cup measure, and a tablespoon measure. Put the large metal spoon in the pot with the soybeans. Leave the tablespoon along with a tablespoon (15 ml) or so of boiled water in the dish. Once this water has cooled to body temperature or below, use the tiny spoon that came with the natto-moto to measure a half spoon of spores, or whatever amount is recommended by the instructions that came with the spores, and add these spores to the water in the dish. Then use the tablespoon to stir the water together with the spores. (Note: The ratio of spores to beans can probably be even lower than this, but it is hard to measure smaller amounts of spores.)

4. Inoculate. Add the hydrated spores to the somewhat-cooled soybeans and mix well using the large metal spoon.

5. Incubate. Place the vessel containing the soybeans in the incubator if it's not already in it. Set it to run for 24 hours at 104°F (40°C), or as close as you can get to this temperature. Make sure the incubator seals well so that your natto won't dry out or get contaminated.

6. After 24 hours, open the incubator and, using a clean spoon, give the natto a stir. If it is not yet sufficiently mucilaginous, incubate it for another 6 hours. Otherwise, move the natto into the small airtight containers, filling the containers as full as possible. Put the containers in the refrigerator for at least a few hours before eating to finalize the fermentation.

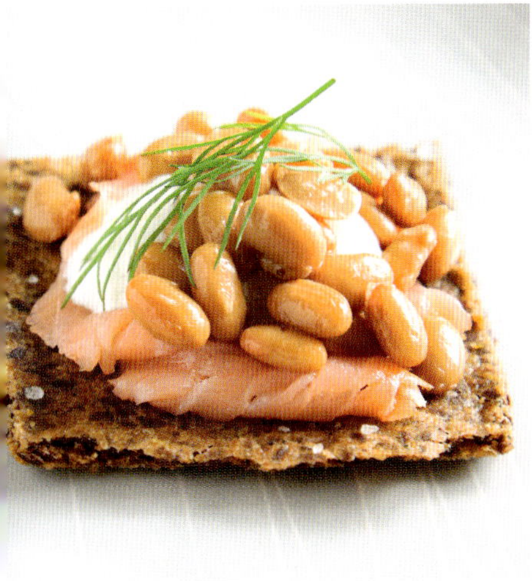

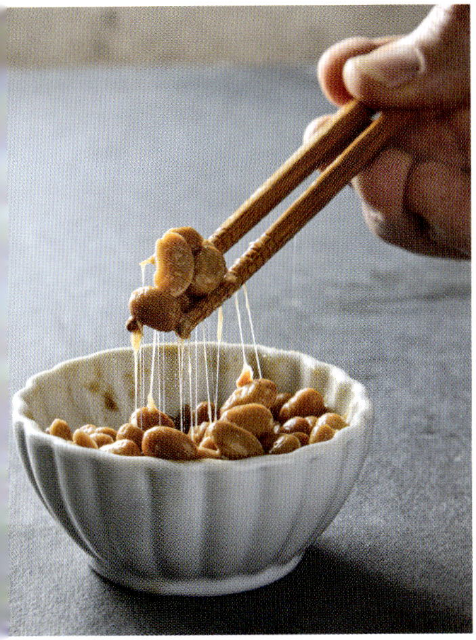

STORAGE

Natto can be stored in the refrigerator for up to a week, or in the freezer for a long time. It is more temperamental than, say, sauerkraut, so be extra sure to use a clean spoon when removing it from its container if you're not using the whole thing.

SERVING

Typically, natto is served over warm rice, with prepared mustard and sweet soy sauce. Other common additions include raw egg yolk and snipped green onion.

But this is just the beginning. Some other possibilities are pictured and described below and can be seen at www.instagram.com/explore/tags/19daysofnatto/.

- Natto makizushi (sushi rolls)
- Natto over rice with soy sauce, egg yolk, avocado, lemon zest, snipped green onions, and shichimi togarashi
- Natto over rice with ikura (salmon eggs), wasabi, snipped green onions, and nasturtium flower
- Sourdough crêpe, fermented beet, crème fraîche, natto, paprika
- "Natto Nachos": corn chips with (fermented) mango salsa, natto, (fermented) jalapeño, crème fraîche, and cilantro
- "La Mancha": sourdough cracker with manchego, gochujang or dry chorizo, shiso leaf, natto, smoked paprika, and olive oil
- "Nattzpacho": gazpacho, natto, cilantro, shichimi togarashi
- "The New England": sourdough cracker with cheddar, apple or pear, kimchi, and natto
- "The Superfood": sourdough cracker with natto, grated fresh turmeric, ground black pepper, fish sauce, and cod liver or cod liver oil

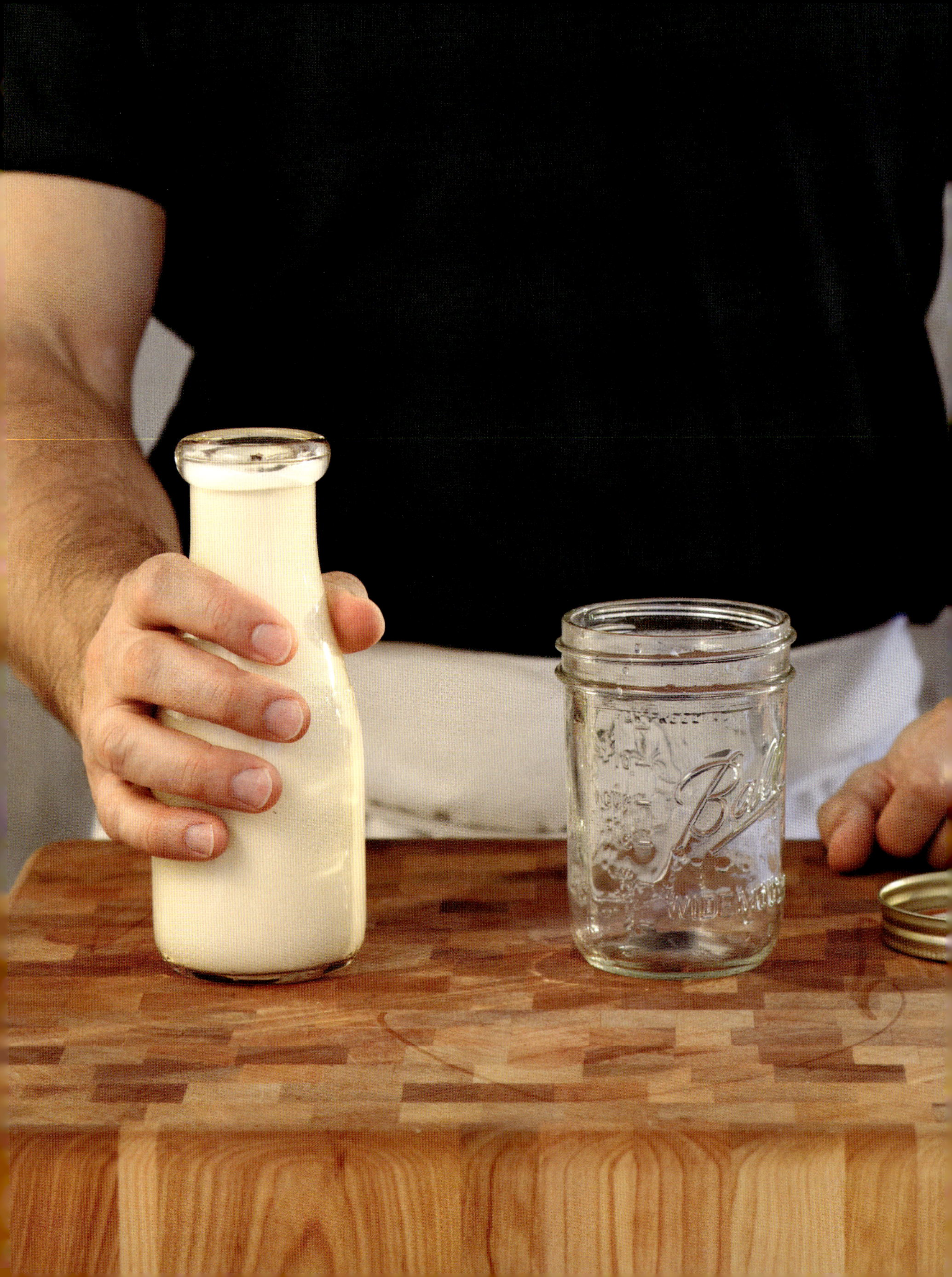

CHAPTER 4

Dairy

In many parts of the world, it's easy to go to the store, buy some milk, bring it home, and put it in the refrigerator, to be consumed over the course of the next week or so. The milk may have been drawn from animals hundreds or thousands of miles away, weeks before it was bought.

This has not always been possible.

A hundred years ago, homes did not have electrically powered refrigerators and freezers. Some homes had iceboxes: insulated boxes kept cool by actual blocks of ice. Iceboxes were neither universal nor convenient, and ice was expensive and perishable.

So in the past, storage of milk was an issue. After several hours at typical room temperatures, fresh milk was no longer fresh, so it was necessary to find ways to extend its life. There are various excellent options, and many of them involve fermentation.

Yogurt

PREP TIME: 30 MINUTES • TOTAL TIME: 12–24 HOURS

It is likely that yogurt originated accidentally in the Middle East more than 4,500 years ago. Options for transporting milk (and other liquids) were limited; putting the milk in animal skins was a good option because the skins were available and waterproof. A plausible scenario: The natural bacteria from an animal skin could have combined with milk, and along with the warm temperatures, could have led to something we would recognize today as yogurt. Once the yogurt culture had found a home in this animal skin, the same skin could be used to make a new batch, or the yogurt itself could be used as a starter.

People have eaten yogurt for millennia; it is a traditional food around the Mediterranean and in western, central, and southern Asia. In recent years, it has found its way to North America, northern Europe, and to parts of East Asia, where consumption of dairy products may not be as widespread.

Yogurt is produced by bacterial fermentation of milk at warm temperatures. The precise collection of bacteria varies somewhat from one sample to another, and different bacteria result in different tastes and textures. It is typically made by heating milk, rendering it more or less sterile; allowing the milk to cool to around 110°F (43°C); then introducing the desired collection of bacteria to the milk and keeping it warm for long enough to allow the bacteria to do their work.

INGREDIENTS

6 tablespoons (90 g) yogurt, as a starter (see page 73)

1 quart (1 L) milk, less 6 tablespoons (90 g)

EQUIPMENT

1-quart (1 L) or two 1-pint (500-ml) mason jar(s)

Medium saucepan

Food thermometer

Incubator big enough to hold all your mason jars (an insulated bag or cooler, a pilot light-style oven that can stay at approximately 110°F [45°C], a food dehydrator with the thermostat set at 110°F [45°C], a multicooker with a "yogurt" mode, or a yogurt maker!)

A few extra mason jars of any size

—

Yield: 1 quart (1 L)

PREPARATION

1. Measure out the yogurt that you're going to use as a starter (a). Put it in the quart jar, or split it equally between the pint jars.

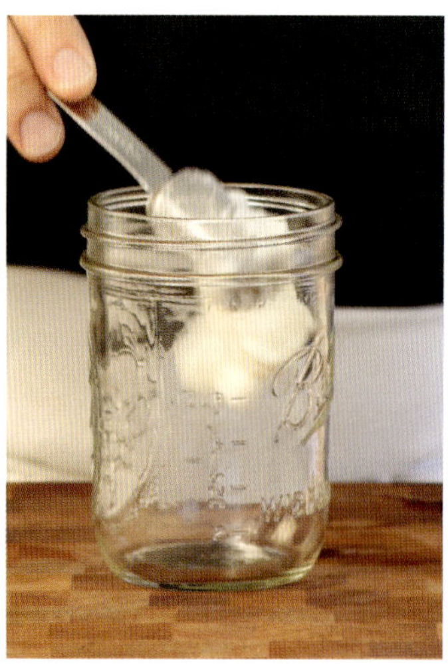

a

2. Heat the milk in the saucepan until it is almost 180°F (80°C) and try to keep it around that temperature for 20 minutes. Take it off the heat and let it cool to 110°F (45°C), or a little warmer. If you are impatient, you may set your pan in cold water or an ice bath, and/or pour the milk into a metal mixing bowl to allow it to cool more quickly.

continued

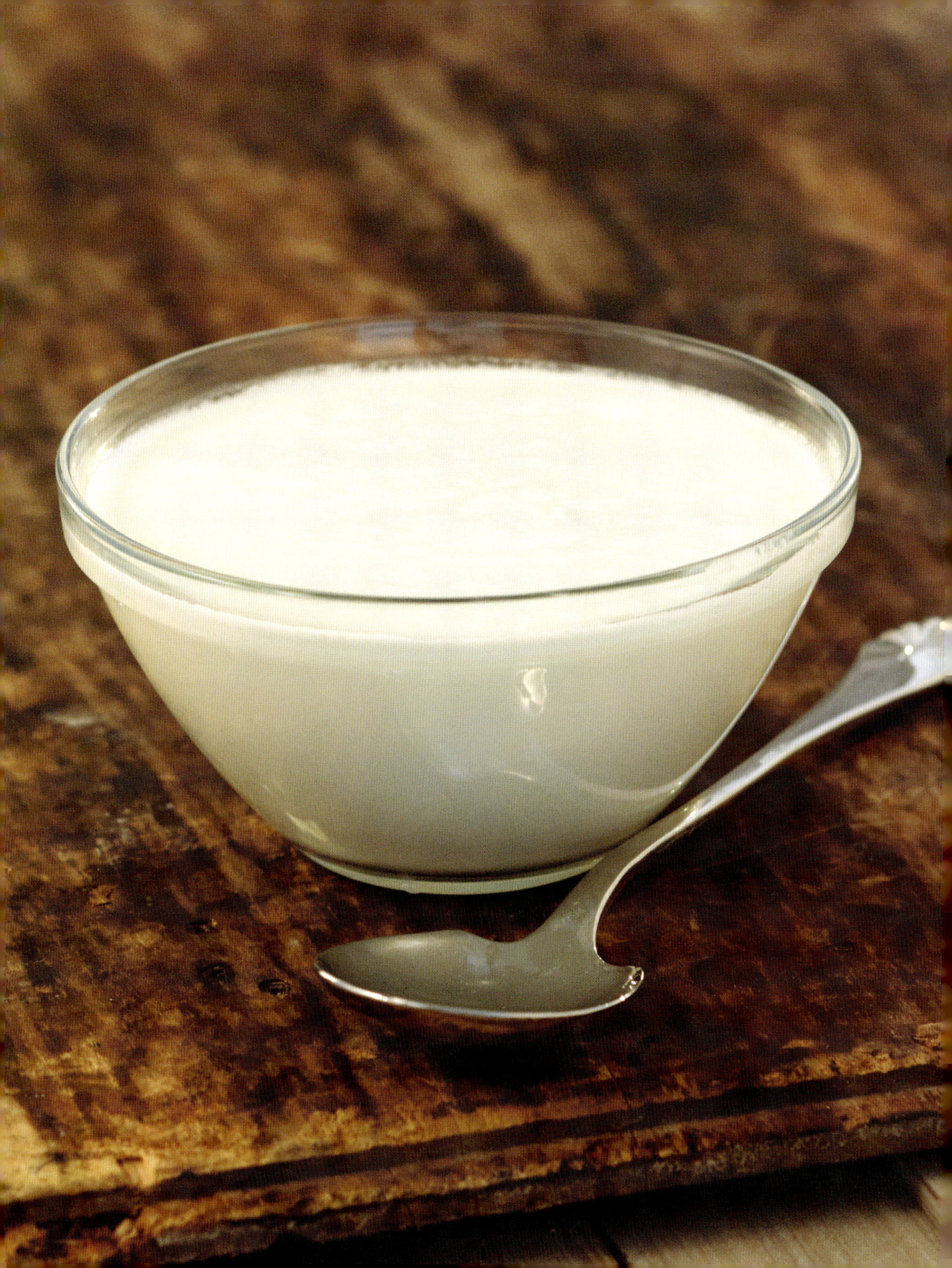

Yogurt *(continued)*

3. Add the milk to the jar, leaving 1 inch (2.5 cm) or so of room at the top (b). Close the jar and shake it so that the yogurt starter mixes well with the milk (c).

4. Put the jar(s) in the warm or insulated incubator you have prepared (d). If your incubator does not have a heat source of its own, fill some of your extra mason jars with hot tap water (130°F–140°F [55°C–60°C]) and put them in the incubator alongside your yogurt jar(s).

5 After 12 to 24 hours, your yogurt will be ready. If you like, put it in the refrigerator, where it will thicken further.

Yogurt will keep in the refrigerator for at least two weeks, and probably longer. After a week or two, it may start to separate, and clear liquid may rise to the top; this is not a problem, and it doesn't mean that the yogurt is spoiling. The clear liquid is yogurt whey, which is explained in the next recipe.

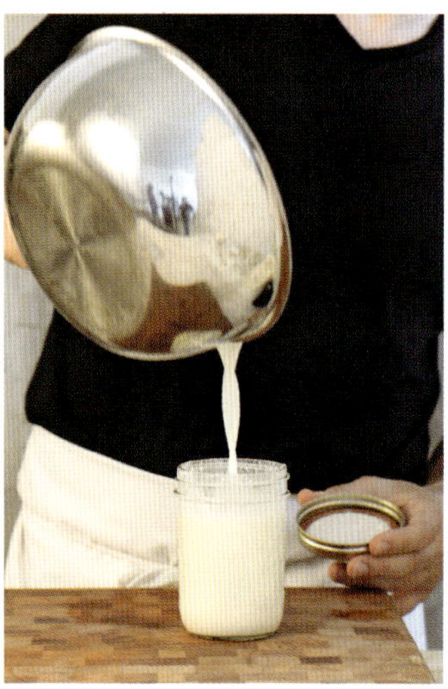

b

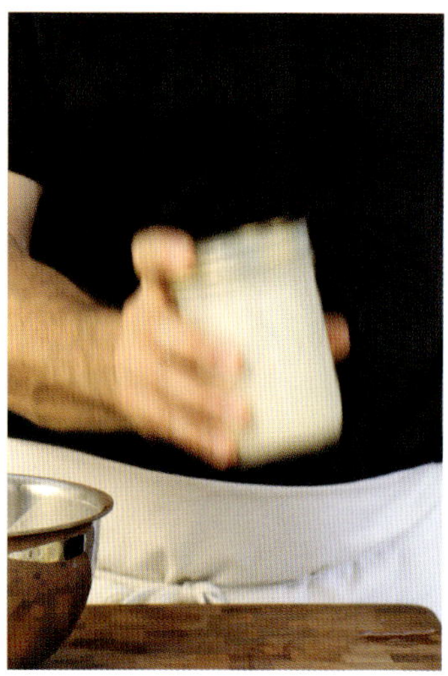

c

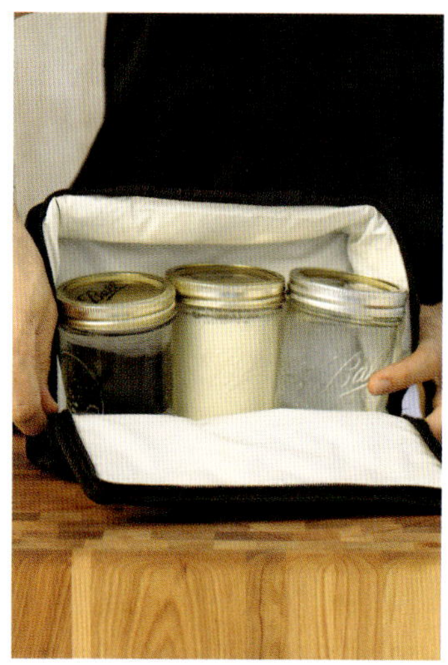

d

YOGURT STARTERS

The better the starter, the better the resulting yogurt. Typically, a portion of an existing batch of yogurt is used as a starter to get the desired bacteria into a new batch. Use homemade yogurt as a starter if you have some. Otherwise, buy the best yogurt you can from the store. Find yogurt that is minimally processed. It should be plain, whole-milk yogurt and as fresh as possible; it should not contain any funny stuff like gelatin or nonfat dry milk powder; and it must contain active yogurt cultures. Read the label carefully. Also, use younger yogurt rather than older. The longer yogurt sits the less active its bacteria will be because once they have finished “eating” the lactose in the yogurt, they have nothing more to eat, and they gradually die off.

Important note: If, and only if, you are starting with raw milk, you may skip the sterilization stage and simply bring the milk up to the favorable temperature range, add your starter, and maintain the temperature. Yogurt made this way will contain a greater variety of beneficial microbes, which is good from a health point of view; however the results will be less predictable, and the yogurt may be thinner than yogurt made from heated milk, so its texture will be less predictable.

CHEESE

Making milk into cheese is yet another way of preserving it, as well as making it easier to transport. Cheese is made by coagulating some of the milk proteins and removing most of the liquid. This liquid is called whey, or cheese whey. Cheese whey is different from yogurt whey (see page 74) because cheesemaking often involves heating the milk, in which case the whey does not contain live bacteria and is therefore not usable as a starter.

Cheeses go through a curding, or curdling, process. Milk is acidulated either by adding an acid, such as lemon juice or vinegar, or by fermenting with specific bacteria. Sometimes it is heated. Whey may be drained off. If you are making curd cheeses such as ricotta, farmers' cheese, Quark, or paneer, you may be done at this point. These cheeses are not much more complicated than curdled milk.

Otherwise, we continue the curdling process with the addition of enzymes, either rennet derived from animal sources or alternative enzymes from plants or fungi. For different results, we use different amounts of enzymes, different ultimate moisture levels, different types of bacteria, more or less salt, more or less aging, sometimes a particular mold, sometimes a coating of wax, and sometimes other sorts of treatments.

This book does not include recipes for cheesemaking, which it is its own entire field of knowledge. It is easy to find articles, books, and even schools dedicated to cheesemaking. See Resources on page 139 for some top recommended reading.

Strained Yogurt and Whey

PREP TIME: 5–20 MINUTES • TOTAL TIME: 4–12 HOURS

When yogurt is left to strain through cheesecloth or muslin, the results are thick, strained yogurt (also known as Greek-style yogurt or *labneh*) and thin yogurt whey, which is the liquid that drains off. Strained yogurt is thicker and richer than regular yogurt and is less inclined to curdle, which makes it usable in some culinary contexts where regular yogurt might not be. Strained yogurt is a delicious spread on bread, for instance, and works nicely to enrich sauces. It is also often served with fruit or honey as a dessert or breakfast.

Yogurt whey is useful in fermenting vegetables and fruits because it is an excellent source of the right sorts of bacteria. (For more instructions on fermenting with whey, see page 44.) It is also a great probiotic drink, pleasantly sour and easy to digest.

INGREDIENTS
1 quart (1 L) plain yogurt (homemade or store-bought)

EQUIPMENT

Fine cheesecloth (find cheesecloth that is not bleached with chlorine)

Large fine-mesh strainer

Mixing bowl or pitcher to suspend the strainer over

Wooden spoon (optional)

—

Yield: Approximately 1 pint (450 g) strained yogurt and 1 pint (500 ml) whey

PREPARATION

1. Moisten the cheesecloth with chlorine-free tap water, and lay it on the inside of the strainer. (By moistening the cheesecloth ahead of time, you minimize the amount of whey that the cheesecloth absorbs.)

2. Put the strainer over the bowl or pitcher.

3. Scoop, spoon, or pour the yogurt into the strainer (a), and let it drain (b).

4. When the yogurt has drained a bit, you may, if you wish, try to tie the ends of the cheesecloth around the handle of the spoon in such a way that it can continue to drain into the bowl or pitcher (c), (d), (e). If you don't do this, then cover the strainer with a plate or something similar to keep foreign objects out of the yogurt.

5. When the yogurt has thickened, put it in a sealed container and refrigerate it; it will continue to thicken as it cools in the refrigerator. Put the whey in the refrigerator, too. Consume them both within a couple of weeks, although they may last longer. When they have started to go bad, you will know because they will get slimy or moldy.

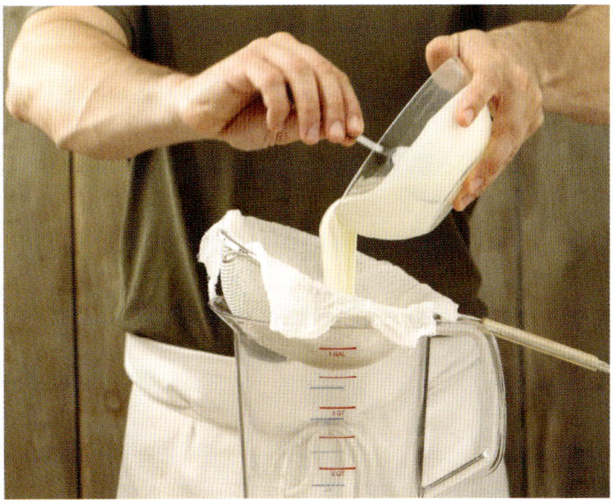

a

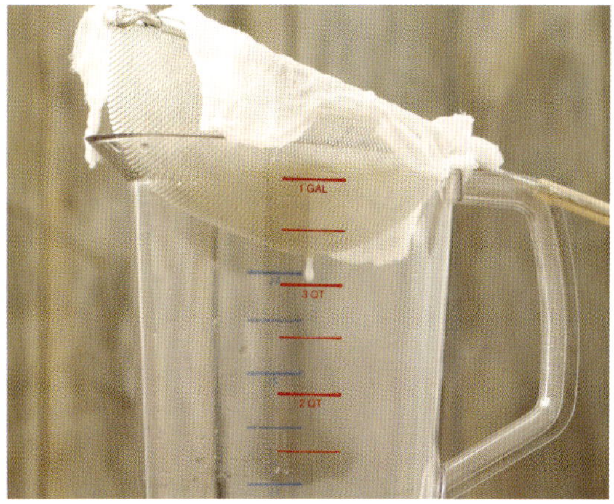

b

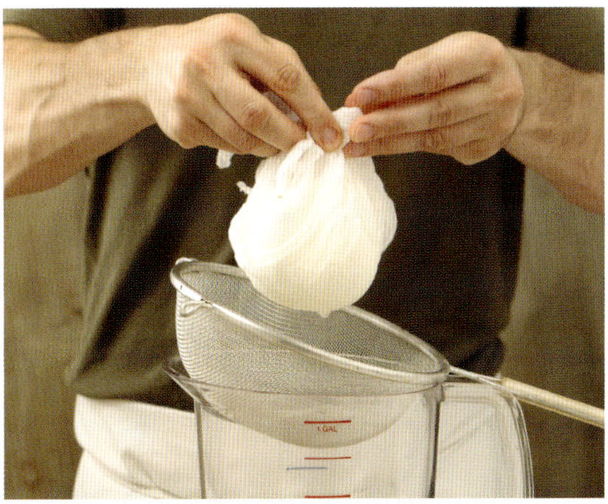

c

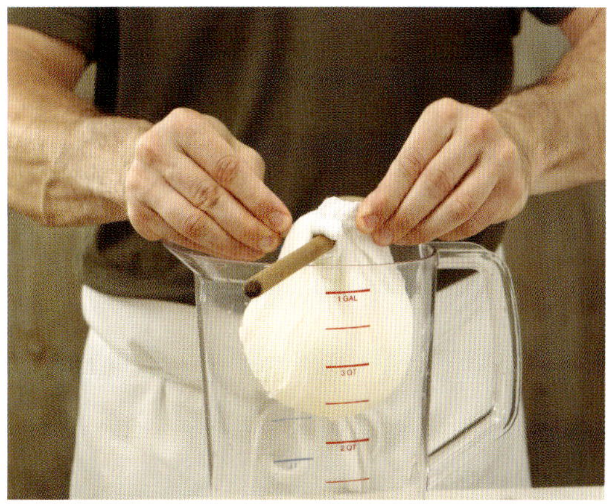

d

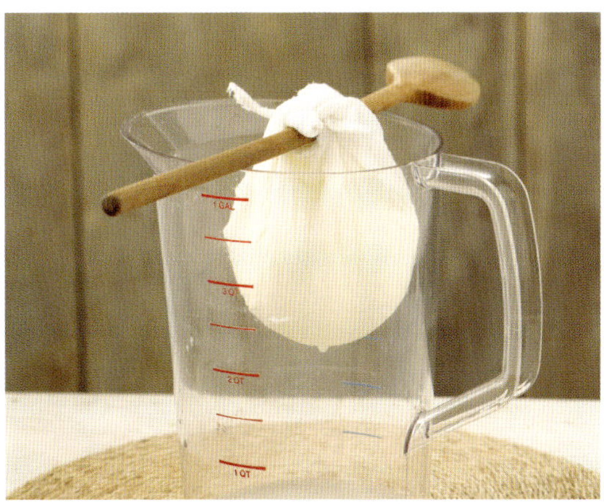

e

Kefir

PREP TIME: 5–20 MINUTES • TOTAL TIME: 12–24 HOURS

Kefir is a fermented milk food that is related to yogurt, though generally thinner in consistency. The origin of kefir is a matter of some speculation. Some accounts hold that it has existed in central Asia since at least 3000 BCE; a legend tells that it was a gift from Allah to Muhammad.

Regardless, the starters necessary to make kefir were guarded by the people of the region until the early twentieth century, at which time a Russian spy supposedly stole some of the starters and brought them to Moscow, whence they spread far and wide. Today, kefir is enjoyed in some of the same places yogurt is. Because of its generally thinner consistency, it is more likely to be consumed as a drink or as a component in a drink, in place of milk, or in a soup. The biggest practical differences between kefir and yogurt are (1) the microbes responsible for kefir are industrious at room temperature, while yogurt's are most productive above about 100°F (40°C); and (2) a kefir starter is a cottage cheese–like collection of globules, referred to as "grains," which is strained out and reused repeatedly.

Kefir grains are combinations of yeasts and bacteria living on a substrate made up of a variety of dairy components. After you use them to start your batch of kefir, you can strain them out and save them to start your next batch. Each time you use them, they grow slightly in size. You can get kefir starters at health food stores, via the Internet, or if you're very lucky, from a friend.

INGREDIENTS

1 quart (1 L) milk, or a little less

1–2 tablespoons (15–30 g) kefir grains

EQUIPMENT

Two 1-quart (1-L) mason jars

Small strainer, ideally sized to the mouth of the mason jar

Mixing bowl or pitcher to suspend the strainer over

Wooden spoon (optional)

—

Yield: 1 quart (1 L)

PREPARATION

1. Fill a jar most of the way with milk, leaving some space at the top (1 inch, or 2.5 cm, is sufficient), and then add the kefir grains (a).

2. Put the lid on the jar and shake it (b).

3. Keep the jar at room temperature for 12 to 24 hours (a little less if your room is warm, perhaps a little more if it's cold). Shake it every few hours, if you think of it.

4. Shake the jar one last time. Set the strainer over the second mason jar, and strain the kefir into it (c), (d). Straining allows you to recover your kefir grains (starter).

5. Put a lid on the jar and store the finished kefir in the refrigerator, where it might keep for months, or on the counter, where it might keep for weeks. At some point, it will start to separate, and eventually, it will get unpleasantly sour and yeasty; it will become unappetizing before it becomes unsafe to eat.

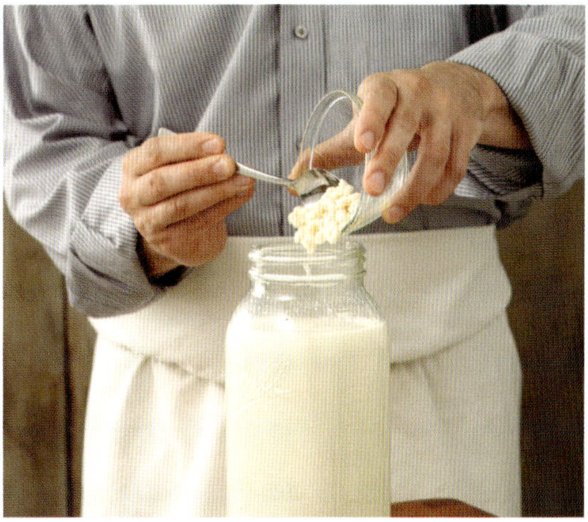

a

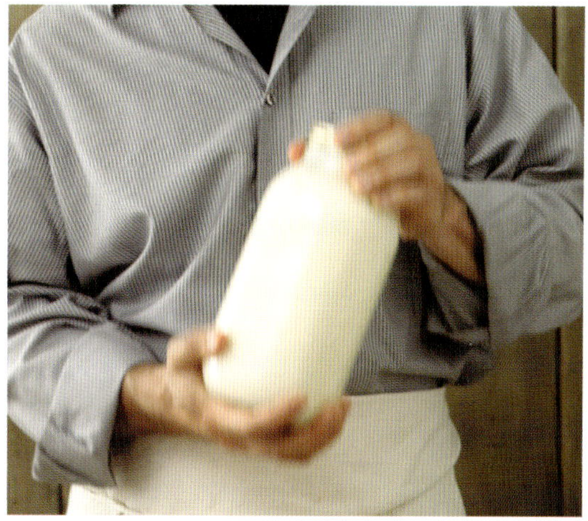

b

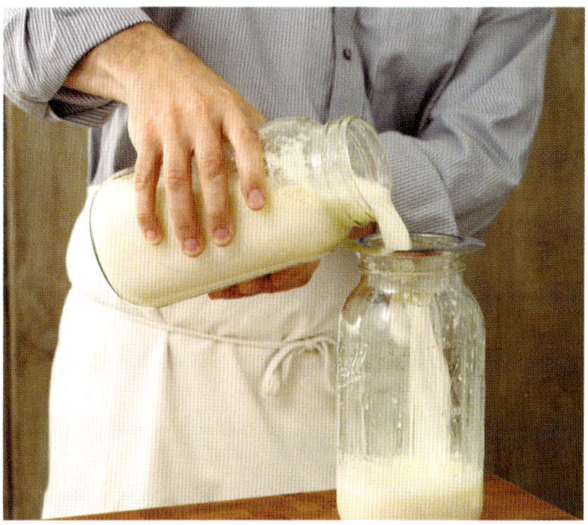

c

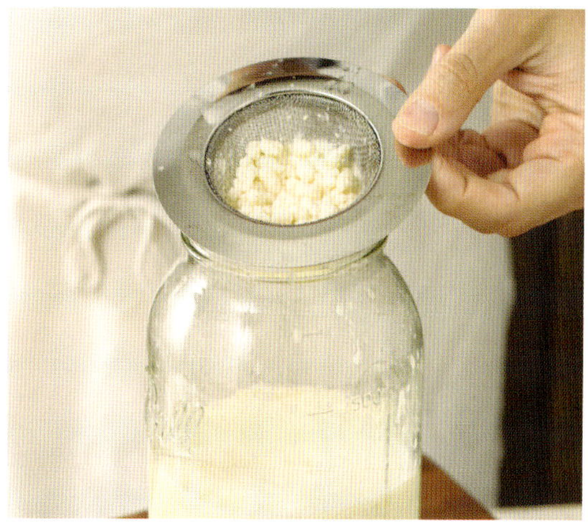

d

6. You may use your kefir grains to start another batch of kefir immediately. Otherwise, rinse them in nonchlorinated water, then store them in a small jar of nonchlorinated water in the refrigerator until the next time you want to use them.

The trickiest part of the kefir-making process is the straining. Especially if you are using unhomogenized milk, it can be difficult to distinguish grains of the kefir starter from globs of milk fat and protein. Shaking the kefir is good because it will break up the globs but not the kefir grains. Also, the sooner you strain the kefir, the less clumpy it will be, and the easier to strain. In any case, it need not be a precise process; nothing bad will happen if, on the one hand, you strain out some of the globs and save it with the starter or, on the other hand, you eat some of the kefir grains. (Just don't eat them all, or you won't be able to make another batch!)

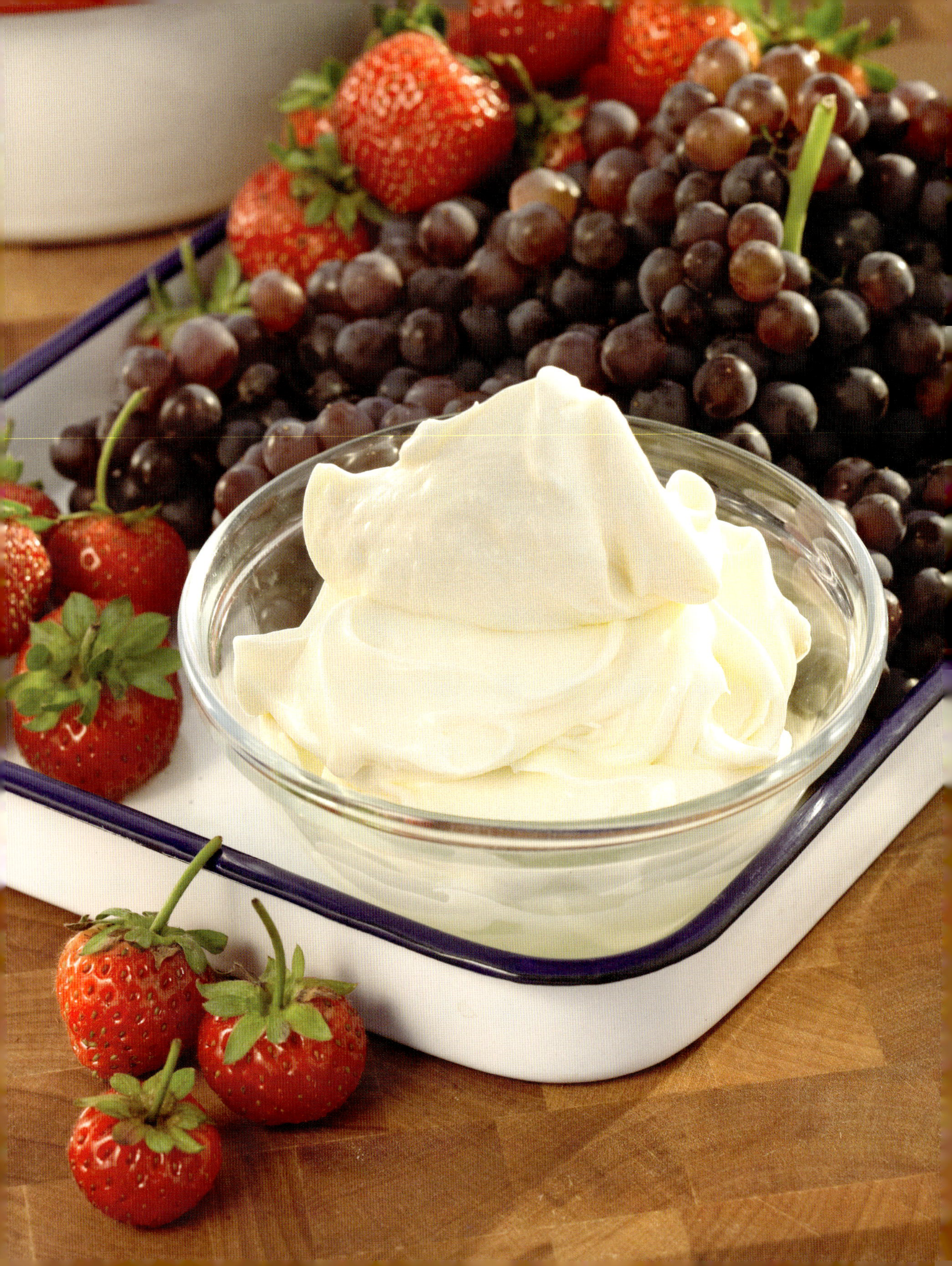

Crème Fraîche

PREP TIME: 10 MINUTES • TOTAL TIME: 12–18 HOURS

Crème fraîche literally means "fresh cream" in French; despite this, crème fraîche is the name given to cream that has been soured.

Originally, crème fraîche was simply unpasteurized cream that had been left out and allowed to ferment through the action of lactic acid bacteria. This same method does not work with pasteurized cream because the lactic acid bacteria are destroyed in the pasteurization process. For those who cannot get unpasteurized cream, an alternative is to start with pasteurized cream, warm the cream, add a starter culture, and let it ferment. Options for starter cultures include yogurt, kefir, and cultured buttermilk (which is available at most supermarkets) (see page 81 for a discussion of buttermilk). Using buttermilk probably gets you closest to what unpasteurized cream would do on its own. Or, if you have a previous batch of homemade crème fraîche, that is an excellent starter!

Crème fraîche typically has a butterfat content of 30 to 40 percent. What is called sour cream in the United States is similar to crème fraîche but is made from a mixture of cream and milk (half-and-half) and typically weighs in at about 18 percent to 20 percent butterfat. The sour cream you buy at the store all too frequently contains thickening and acidifying agents, and sometimes flavorings of various sorts. You can also buy "lite" sour cream, which has less fat and more additives, and even nonfat sour cream, which has no fat and still more additives. Store-bought sour cream, like store-bought crème fraîche, may have been pasteurized after fermentation, in which case it can't be used as a starter. If you have bought some sour cream or crème fraîche from the store and you're not sure about it, don't use it as a starter; it's easier to use buttermilk or yogurt.

Making sour cream at home is a bit harder than making crème fraîche, and the result is a bit less luxurious, so why not make crème fraîche? But if you would like to make sour cream, it's best to try to regulate its temperature as you would when making yogurt.

You can make crème fraîche pretty much the way you make yogurt (see page 70), except that you can use different starters, and it is not as picky about temperature. It's possible to make it in a warm room without using any insulated or heated containers. If you can't get unpasteurized cream, pasteurized cream will do, with a starter. Ultra-pasteurized cream works fine for me, too, although some people who try to use it report problems.

continued

Crème Fraîche *(continued)*

INGREDIENTS
12–13 ounces (350–400 ml) unpasteurized cream

3 tablespoons (45 g) yogurt, kefir, or cultured buttermilk as a starter, if using pasteurized cream; starter is optional if using raw cream

EQUIPMENT
1-pint (500-ml) mason jar

—

Yield: 1 pint (450 g)

PREPARATION

1. If using a starter, measure out the amount you're going to use. Put it in the mason jar.

2. Add the cream to the jar, leaving 1 inch (2.5 cm) or so of room at the top. Close the jar and shake it so that the starter mixes well with the cream.

3. Place the jar somewhere warm for 12 hours or overnight. Check the cream. If it has not yet thickened, leave it for another 6 hours.

4. When it has thickened, store it in the refrigerator, where it will keep for a week or two.

Crème fraîche is great for cooking because it won't curdle the way cream sometimes does when you heat it or when you add an acid like lemon juice or vinegar.

STORE-BOUGHT CRÈME FRAÎCHE

Be aware that store-bought crème fraîche has often been pasteurized after fermentation, so its bacteria have been killed. It is not useful as a starter, and it has lost its probiotic benefits. If it doesn't say "live cultures" on the packaging, then it's likely that it has been pasteurized.

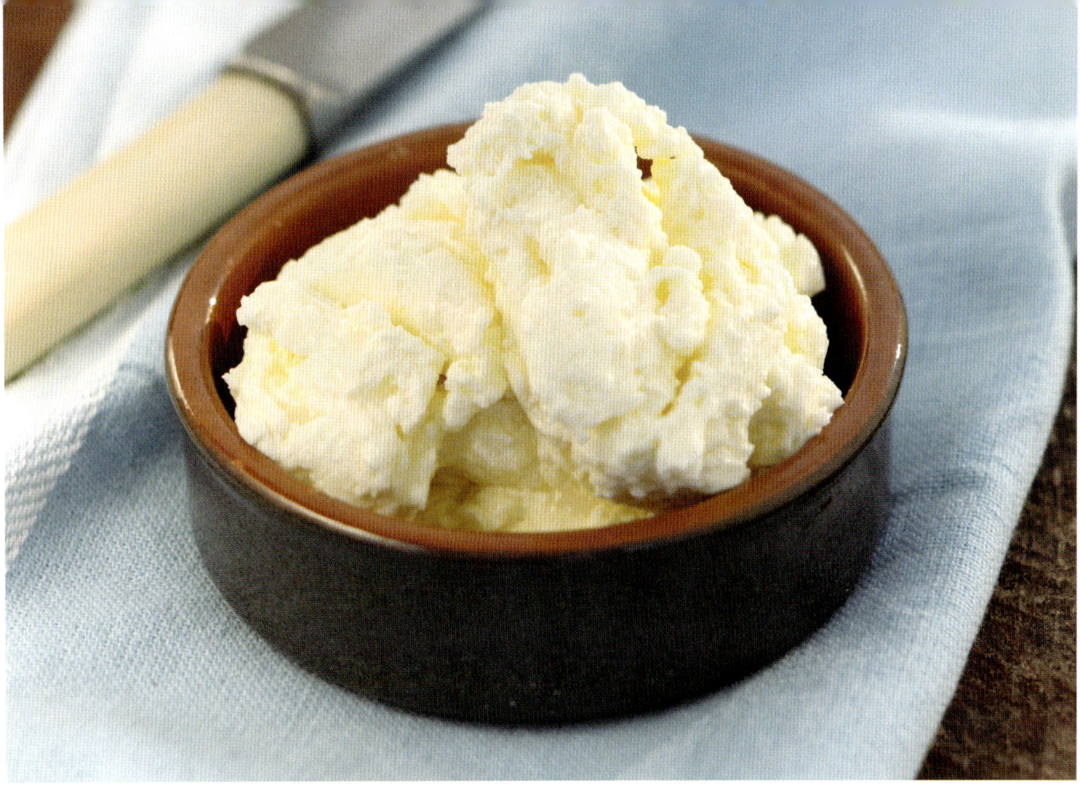

Butter and Buttermilk

PREP TIME: 10–15 MINUTES • TOTAL TIME: 10–15 MINUTES

Making cream into crème fraîche is one way to preserve it. By making it more acidic, you are making it less prone to spoilage. Another way to preserve cream is to turn it into butter, thus removing most of the water and carbohydrates from it, leaving a little protein and a lot of fat. In fact, you can get the best of both worlds by making crème fraîche and then turning it into butter!

When you make butter from unfermented cream, you get what is called sweet cream butter. When you make it from fermented cream (like crème fraîche), using the same process, you get cultured butter.

Making butter is simple: you put cream in a jar, and shake the jar until the cream turns into butter. It's even easier if you have children: hand the jar over to them! You can also use a blender, mixer, or food processor if you have one.

When you are done, you will have butter, and you will have some residual liquid. This residual liquid is true buttermilk. The buttermilk you get from making cultured butter is more interesting than the buttermilk you get from making sweet cream butter: it has more flavor, is more acidic, and contains live cultures. Either way, genuine buttermilk is fat free, or pretty close to it, because the fat is in the butter.

continued

Butter and Buttermilk *(continued)*

INGREDIENTS
Cream or cultured cream (crème fraîche, for example)

Ice water

Sea salt (optional)

EQUIPMENT
A couple of mason jars

Blender, food processor, stand mixer, or hand-held electric mixer (optional)

Small bowl

Medium bowl

Wooden spoon

Cutting board (with a channel, if available) (optional)

—

Yield: Varies

PREPARATION

1. Put the cream in a mason jar (a), close the lid tightly, and shake it until it becomes solid (b). Alternatively, use your equipment to blend it until it solidifies (c).

2. Pour off the liquid into a small bowl (d).

3. Add some ice or ice water to your butter (e), and agitate it again (f). This will help draw off more liquid.

4. Using a wooden spoon or other instrument of your choice, transfer the butter to a medium bowl or turn it out onto a cutting board.

5. Massage the butter with the wooden spoon to remove even more residual liquid (g). The more liquid you can remove, the better your butter will keep.

6. Before you're done massaging it, add salt to taste, if desired.

7. Refrigerate your butter. Optionally, once it has chilled and firmed up, massage it again to get more of the liquid out.

LAB NOTES

If you decide to make cultured butter, you can use partially fermented cream. So, for instance, you can follow the procedure for making Crème Fraîche (page 80), but you don't have to let it ferment for quite as long.

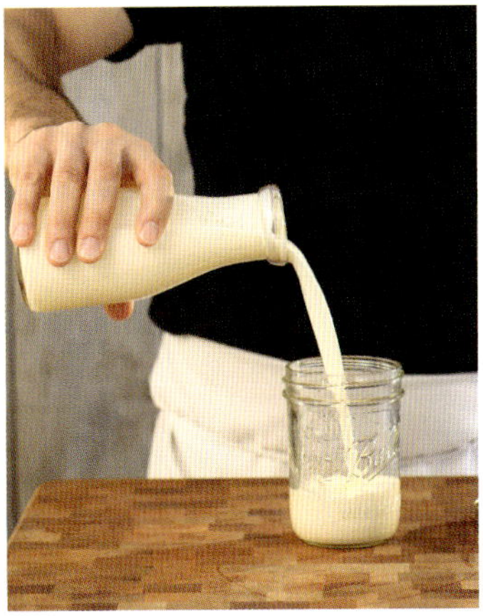

a

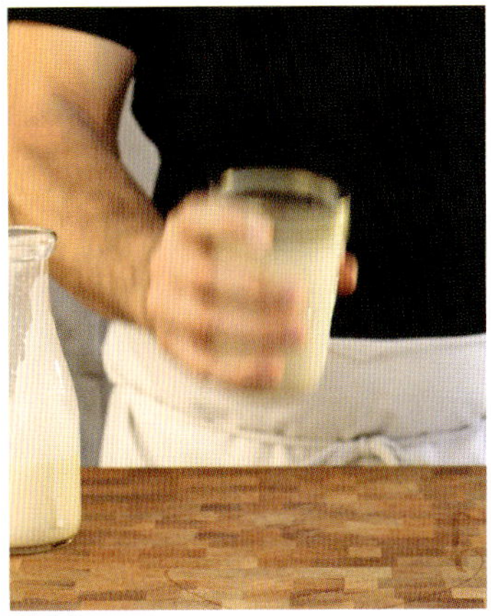

b

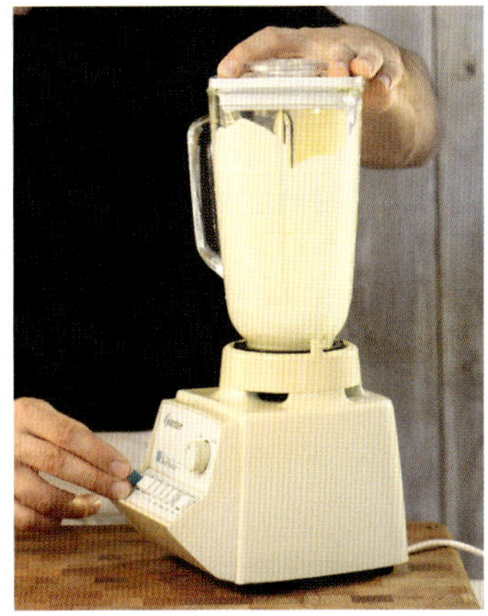

c

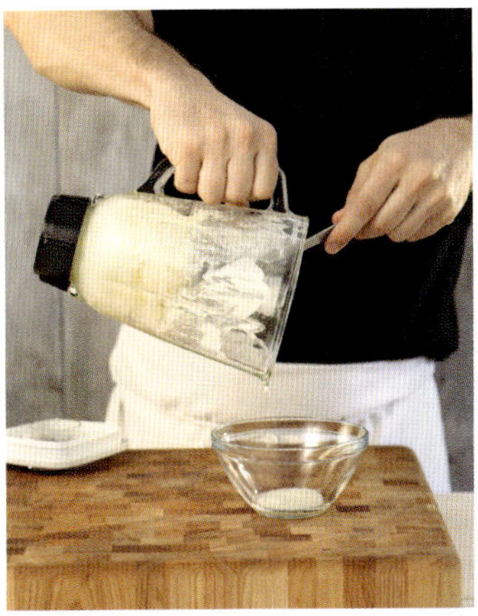

d

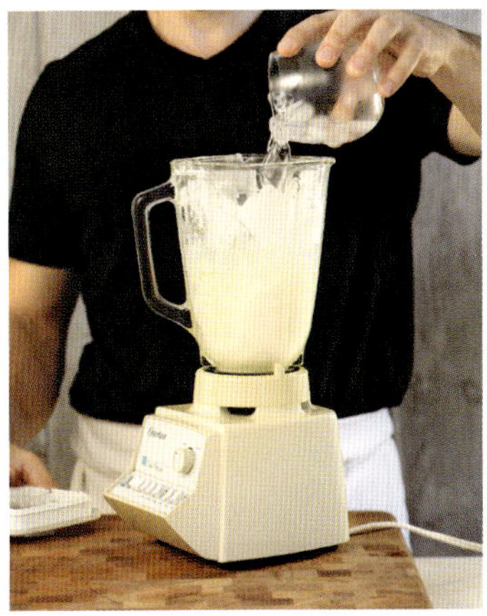

e

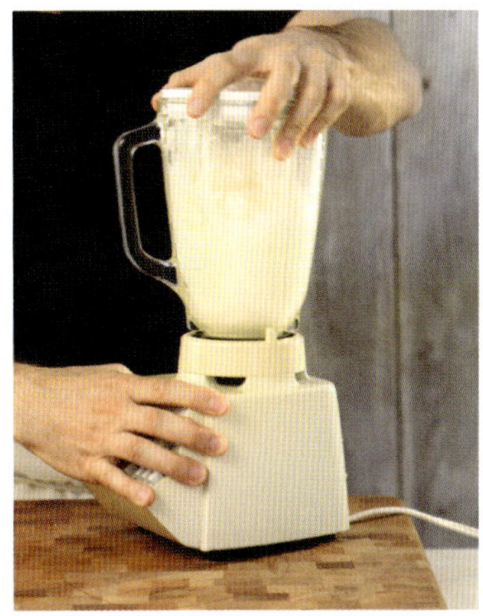

f

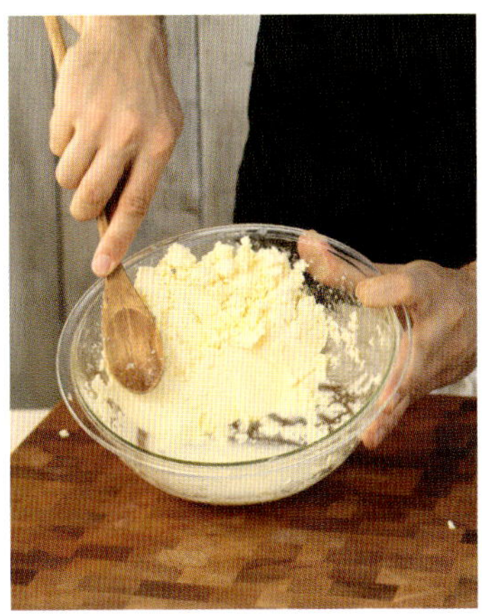

g

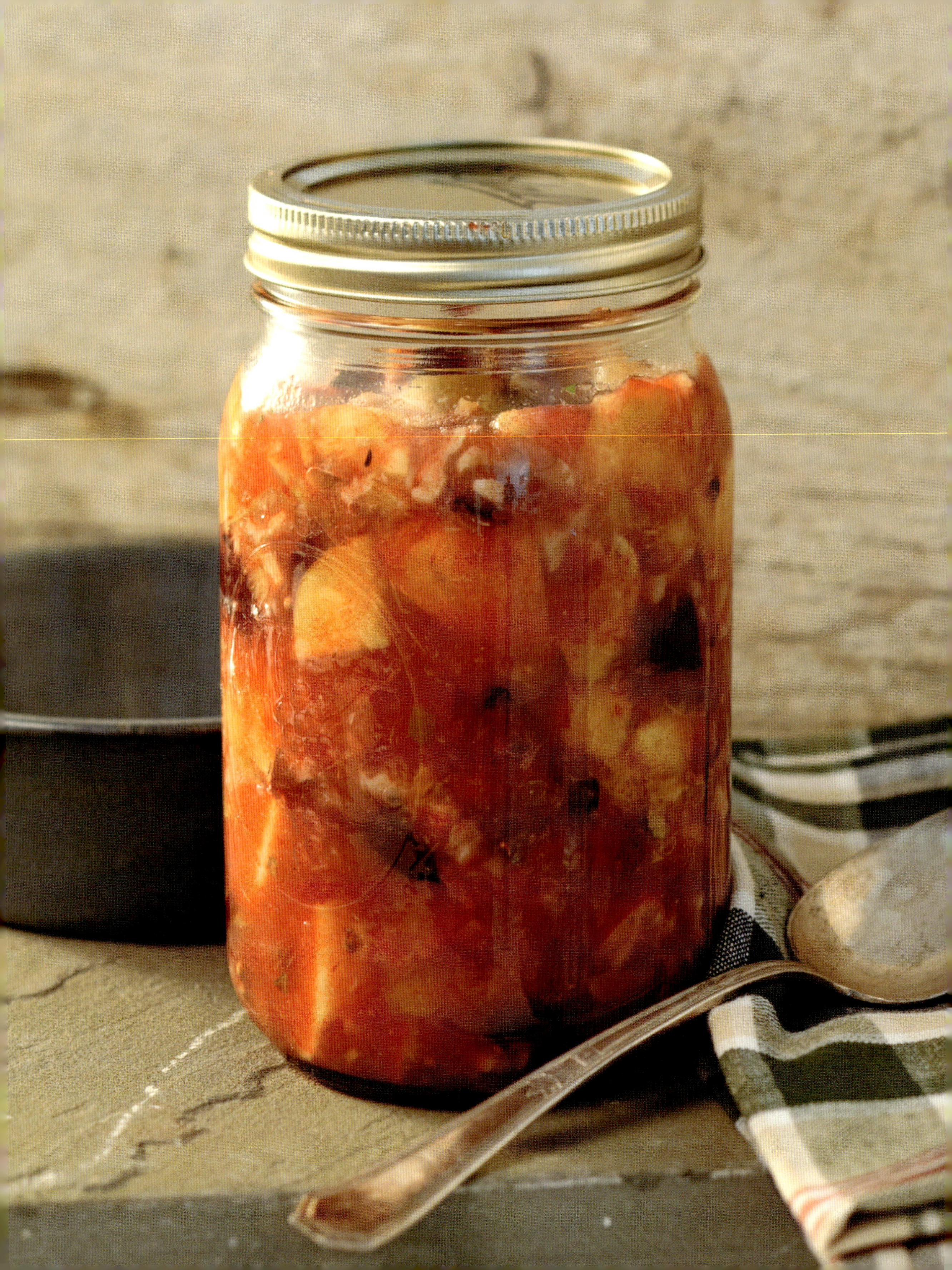

CHAPTER 5

Fermented Fruit Condiments

Fruit, especially soft fruit, has a short shelf life at room temperature. Even in the refrigerator, it loses its appeal pretty quickly. And when we grow it, soft fruit has the infuriating habit of becoming ripe all at once. By the end of summer, we may become blasé about perfectly ripe peaches, but come February, we may crave them. And the peaches in the supermarket will probably not be as good as the ones we found at the farmers' market in the summer.

Fermenting fruit allows us to preserve the summer's bounty until a time when we can appreciate it again. Fermentation also allows us to develop sweet-and-sour flavors that might be better accompaniments for savory dishes, say, than the unrelenting delicious sweetness of fresh fruit.

Many soured foods we eat today can trace their roots to traditional bacterially fermented foods. We have seen that this is the case for vegetables and for dairy; it is also the case for fruit.

Preserved Lemons and Limes

PREP TIME: 10 MINUTES • TOTAL TIME: 6 MONTHS

When preserved, especially when preserved with spices, lemons and limes take on a complex, deep set of flavors. In addition, they can keep for months or even a year or longer, tasting more and more interesting as time goes on.

Preserved lemons are important in North African and Middle Eastern cooking. Limes preserved in the same way play a role in Southeast Asian cuisine. Either, or a mixture of both, can add a unique flavor to ceviche or cocktails. And in fact, squeezing a wedge or two of preserved citrus into a glass with some ice and a little sugar gives you a fantastic summer drink—nature's own sports drink, with electrolytes and quick carbohydrates but none of the preservatives or colorings of commercial sports drinks: the ultimate lemonade.

Nonorganic citrus fruits accumulate pesticides in their rinds, so here it is very important to use organic lemons and limes or lemons and limes from your own trees if you are lucky enough to have them.

INGREDIENTS

1½ pounds (0.75 kg) lemons and/or limes (about 5 or 6 lemons or 8 to 10 limes, depending on size), at room temperature

¼ cup (60 g) sea salt (see page 34)

Assorted spices of your choice: a cinnamon stick, a bay leaf, a few cloves, a few peppercorns, a handful of coriander seeds, or a shake of "pickling spice" (optional)

1 or 2 additional lemons, for juice

EQUIPMENT

Large cutting board (wood is ideal)

A large knife (a chef's knife is ideal)

1-pint (500-ml) mason jar with a tight-fitting lid

—

Yield: 1 pint (500 ml)

PREPARATION

1. Take the lemons and/or limes out of the refrigerator an hour ahead of time to bring them to room temperature.

2. If they are waxed, or if you're not sure, blanch them in boiling water for 30 seconds, then take them out and let them cool.

3. Soften the fruit by rolling them on the counter under your palm, exerting some pressure, but not so much that the rinds split (a), (b).

continued

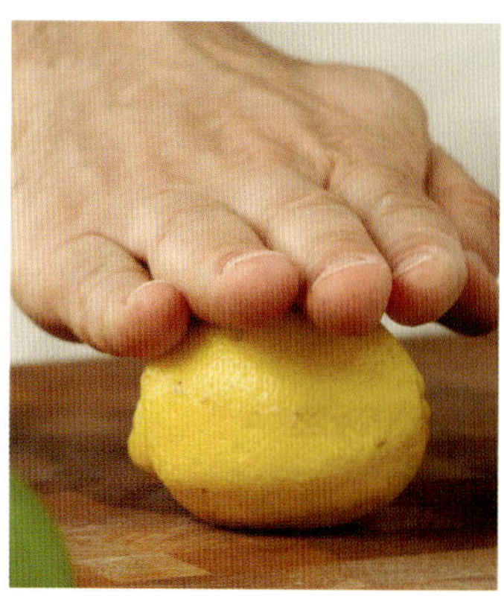

a

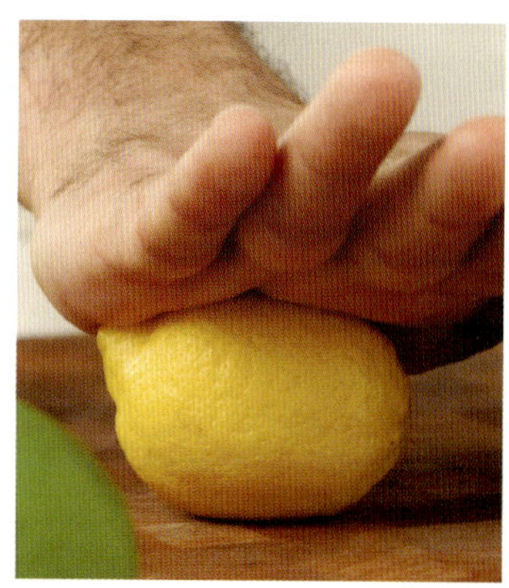

b

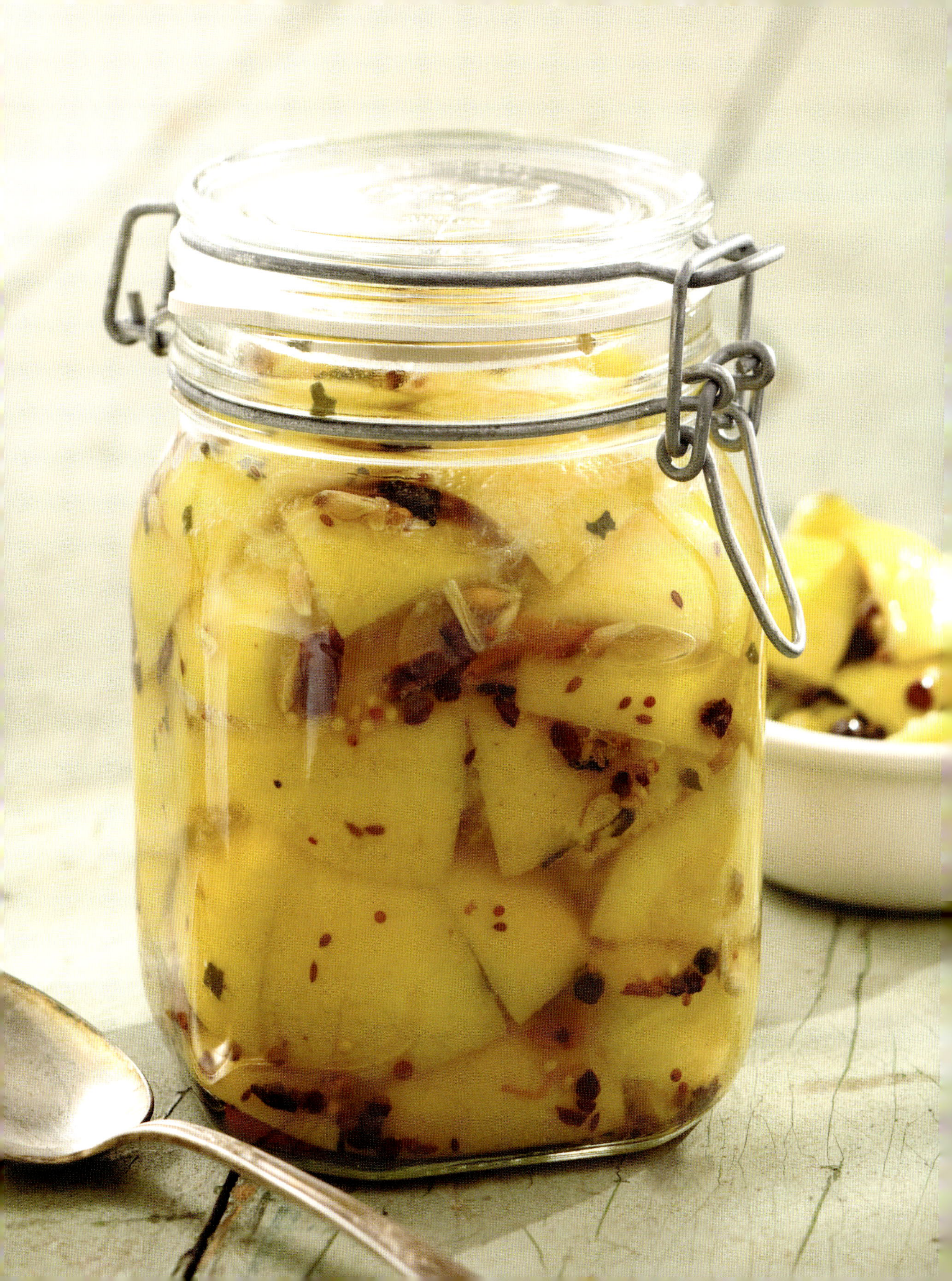

Preserved Lemons and Limes *(continued)*

4. Cut each lemon or lime along its equator (c). Then cut each hemisphere into four wedges (d); alternatively, make these cuts three-quarters of the way through but not all the way. Discard the seeds.

5. Put some salt in the bottom of the jar (e), add some spices, if using, and add a fruit's worth of wedges. Pack down firmly (f). Repeat this, layer by layer, until everything is in the jar, or the jar is nearly full (g). If the released juice does not cover the fruit, juice 1 or 2 additional fruit and add their juice to the jar. Close the jar, leaving 1 inch (2.5 cm) of headroom at the top.

6. Store the jar at room temperature, out of direct sunlight. For the first week, open the jar every day and pack it down so that the liquid rises to cover. The fruit start to change character after a week or two. Left at room temperature, they will continue to deepen in flavor for a year or more. Put them in the refrigerator at any time to slow their progress.

Serving Ideas for Preserved Citrus

- Mince your preserved lemons and use them in cold salads: cucumber, cucumber-yogurt, tuna, potato. Or chop them fine or purée them and mix them with olive oil for a great salad dressing.
- Slice preserved lemons very thin, and serve them with grilled fish. Or serve them with smoked fish and crème fraîche for a trio of preserved foods!
- Finely mince preserved lemons, combine with freshly ground pepper, and rub under the skin of a whole chicken and inside the body cavity before roasting.
- Use preserved lemon in moderation in a tagine or stew, for a deep citrus flavor.
- In Vietnam, there is a salty drink made with ice, preserved lemon, water or carbonated water, and sugar to taste. The same drink works great with limes, too, or a combination of lemons and limes, or probably with any other citrus. Once you try this, you won't want to go back to regular lemonade.

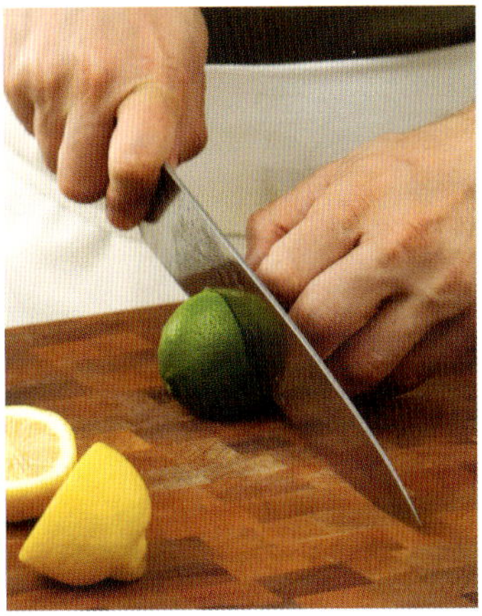

c

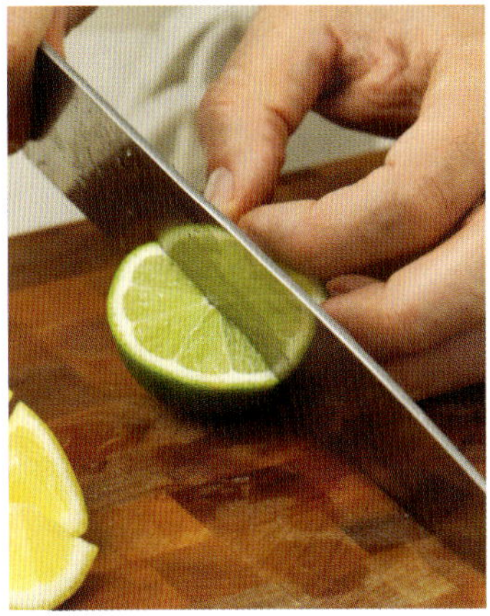

d

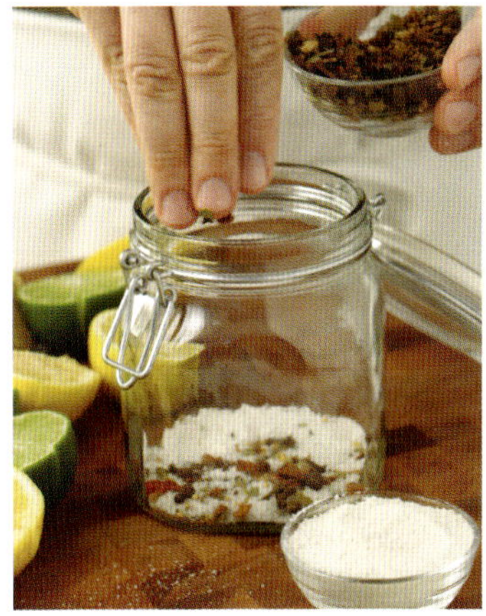

e

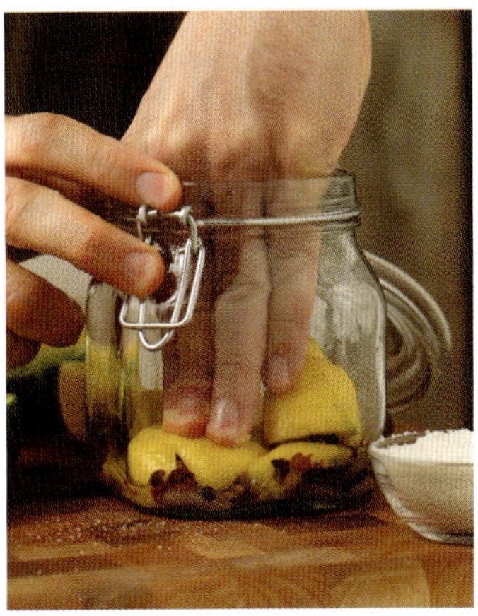

f

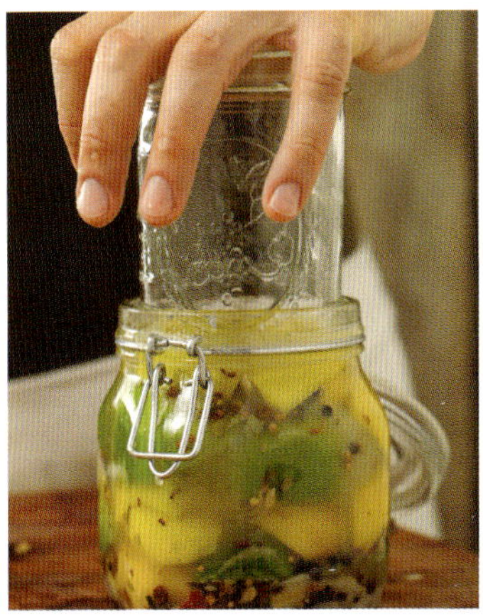

g

LAB NOTES

A little white stuff may grow on the top of the lemons or limes, especially if the juice is low. This is not a problem; simply skim it off, and add more juice. If, however, a lot of fuzzy mold grows, then you should probably throw away your batch and start over.

Other citrus can be fermented, too. Meyer lemons, grapefruit, kumquats, and yuzu are great candidates. Oranges, especially sweet ones, don't work quite as well because of their high sugar content. Remember to find pesticide-free citrus, if you can—it is especially important here, because any pesticide on the rind will permeate the preserved fruit.

Peach and Plum Chutney with Preserved Lime

PREP TIME: 15 MINUTES • OTAL TIME: 4 DAYS

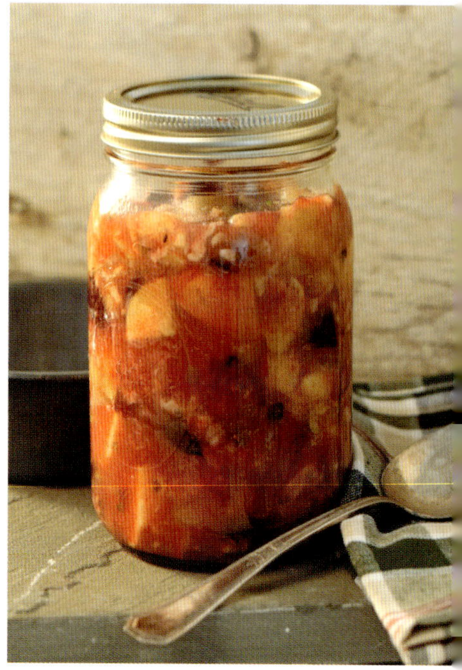

Before refrigeration was widespread, and before canning was understood, people used fermentation to preserve all sorts of foods, including chutneys. These foods developed a distinctive sweet-and-sour flavor.

Today's chutneys are usually preserved with vinegar rather than fermentation. There's nothing really wrong with this, but vinegar-preserved foods don't provide the same health benefits that fermented foods do.

Try this recipe as a side with grilled meats or vegetables: a pork chop, a ham, some swordfish, or a portobello mushroom. You can also mix this chutney into your yogurt for breakfast or a snack, or put it all together in the blender for a great smoothie (add water to thin it out if you like).

INGREDIENTS

Several peaches and plums (approximately 1½ pounds [0.75 kg] total)

A few wedges preserved lime (page 86)

Half a handful chopped walnuts

1 tablespoon (about 6 g) mixed spices, such as cinnamon, cloves, and peppercorns

2 tablespoons (30 ml) yogurt whey

Salt to taste

EQUIPMENT

Large cutting board (wood is ideal)

Large knife (a chef's knife is ideal)

Large mixing bowl

1-quart (1-L) mason jar

—

Yield: a bit less than 1 quart (1 L)

PREPARATION

1. Chop the peaches and plums to the desired size, removing the pits (a), (b).

2. Mince the preserved lime (c).

3. Place all the ingredients into the bowl and mix well (d).

4. Transfer the mixture into the jar, and pack down (e). If the juices are insufficient to cover the chutney, add nonchlorinated water until everything is covered, leaving 1 inch (2.5 cm) of headroom.

5. Close the jar lid tightly, and store at room temperature. Open the jar a couple of times a day to relieve pressure.

6. After 2 to 3 days, when the product is slightly fizzy, put it in the refrigerator.

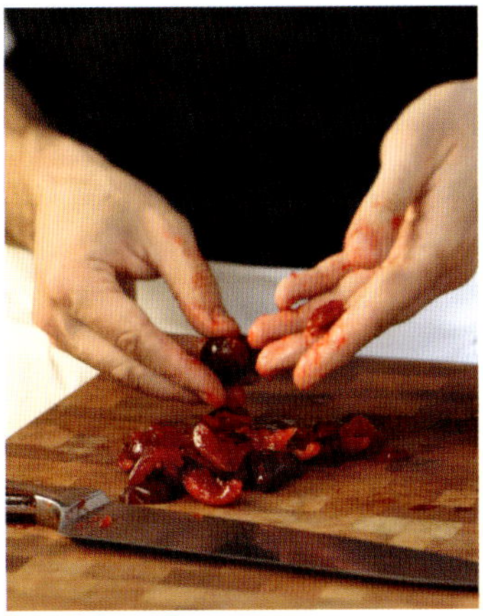

a

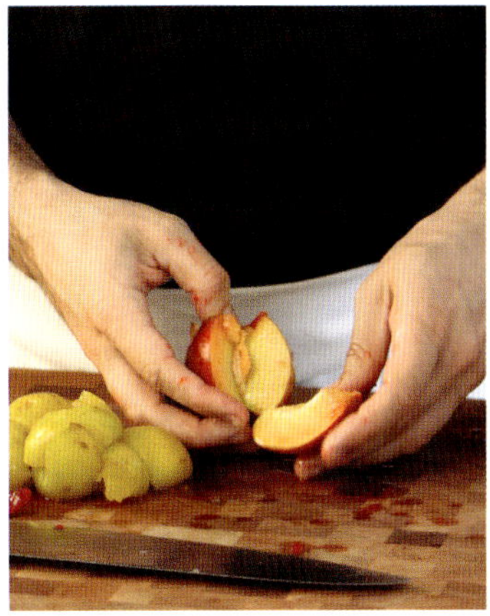

b

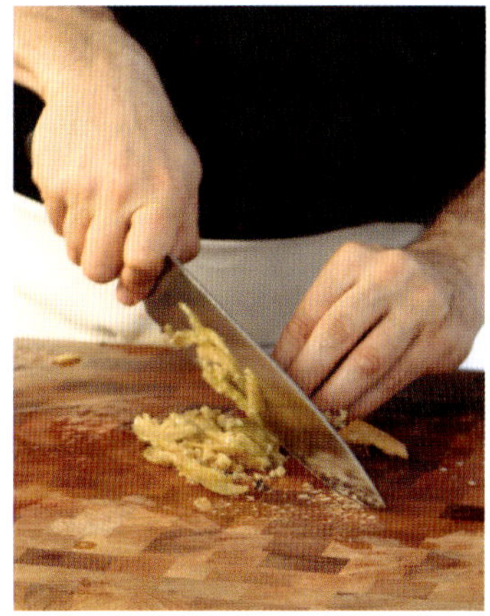

c

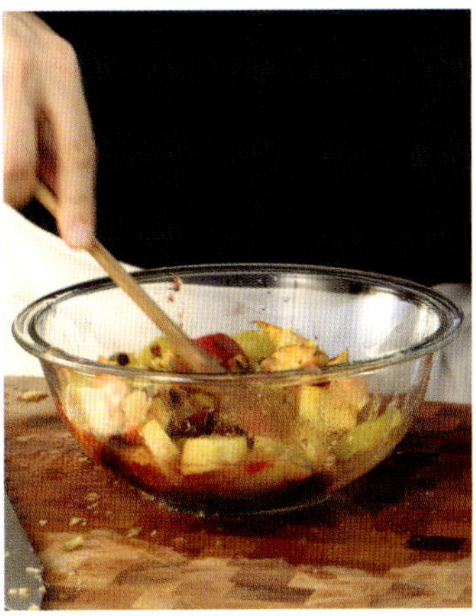

d

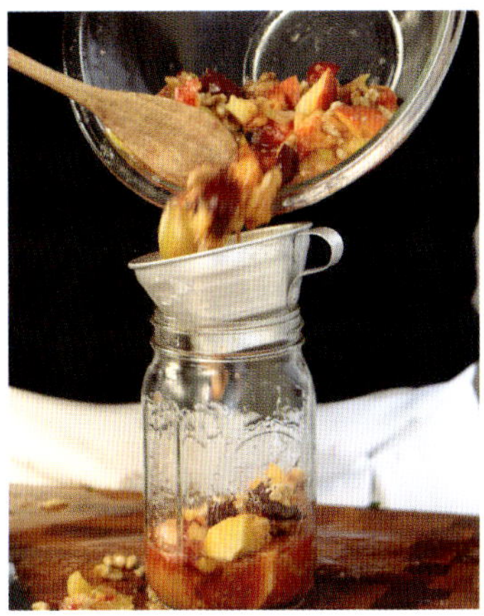

e

LAB NOTES

- Pressure can build up, so be a little bit careful when opening the jar. You may want to do it over the sink!
- Many variations are possible. One option is to cut apples, pears, or Asian pears into cubes, and use those instead of the softer fruit.
- The chutney will keep in the refrigerator for a month or more.

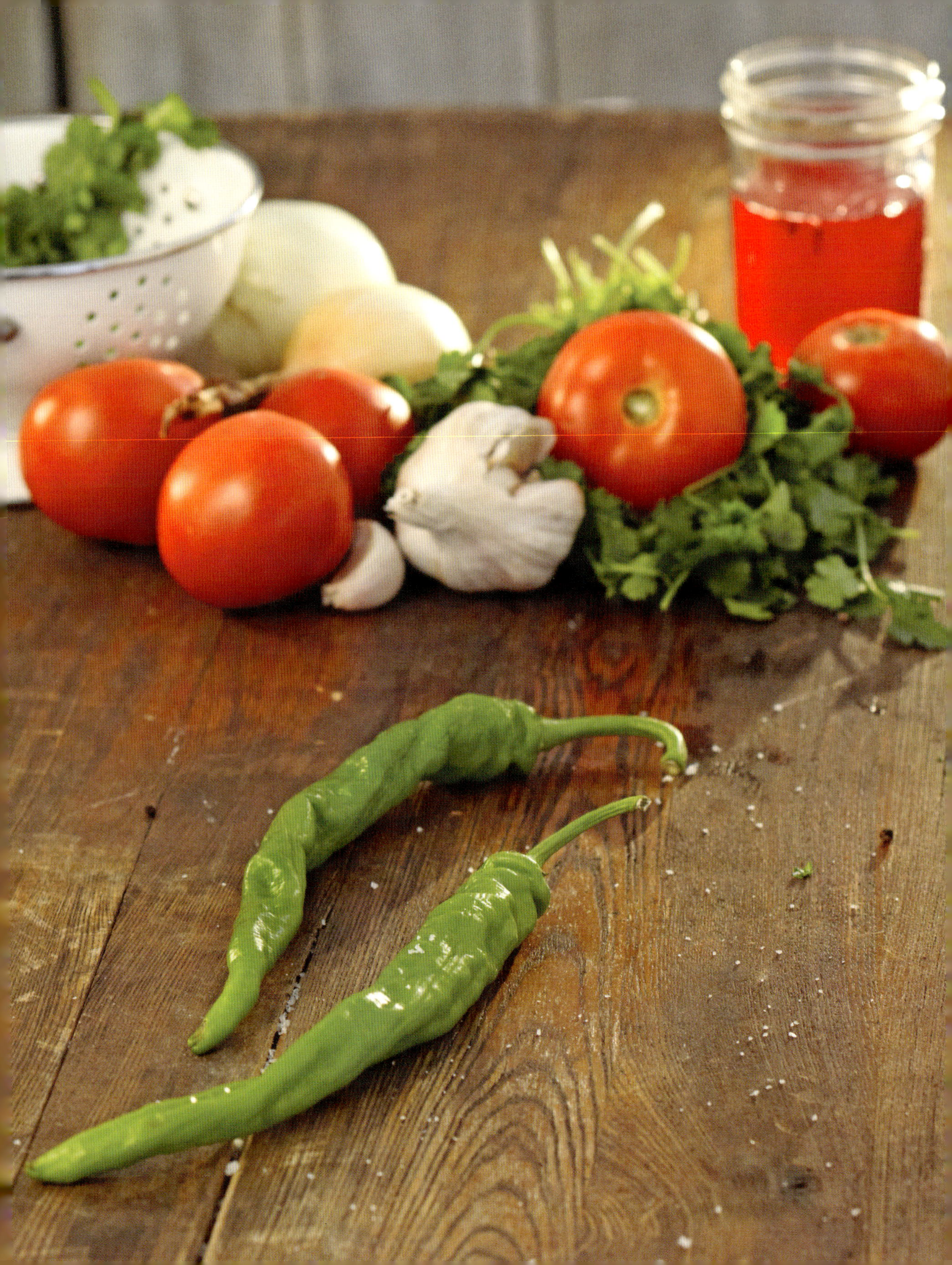

Pico de Gallo

PREP TIME: 25 MINUTES • TOTAL TIME: 3–5 DAYS

Pico de gallo means "beak of the rooster" in Spanish. It is a condiment made with tomatoes, onions, peppers, herbs, and other flavorings. In North America, it is often referred to as "salsa." I prefer to call it "pico de gallo" because "salsa" is a very general term—it translates as simply "sauce."

This recipe requires sauerkraut juice, ideally from a batch of your own sauerkraut (page 39). If you plan to do a lot of fermenting, it's good to always have some sauerkraut on hand.

Tomato skins and cores can be bitter, so I remove them here. If you prefer to leave them in, that's fine, too; and it makes the recipe simpler and quicker.

INGREDIENTS

6 medium tomatoes

1 large onion

½ bunch cilantro

6 cloves garlic

Hot peppers, to taste

1½ cups (350 ml) sauerkraut juice (page 39), from a batch of sauerkraut you have made (requires prior planning)

Salt and pepper to taste

EQUIPMENT

Large stockpot

Ice

Mixing bowl

Paring knife

Tongs or a large slotted spoon

Large knife (a chef's knife is ideal)

Large cutting board (wood is ideal)

1-quart (1-L) mason jar

—

Yield: a bit less than 1 quart (1 L)

PREPARATION

1. Fill the stockpot with water and bring it to a boil.

2. Prepare an ice bath in the mixing bowl.

3. Cut an "X" on the top of each tomato with the paring knife (a).

4. Using tongs, put the tomatoes in the boiling water for approximately 30 seconds, all at once or in batches, until the skin starts to peel (b), and then immediately immerse them in the ice bath (c). This will make them easier to peel.

5. Peel the tomatoes (d), remove their cores (e), and use your fingers to remove some or all of the seeds, so that you are left mostly with the flesh.

6. Chop the tomatoes and all of the other solid ingredients, and add them to the mixing bowl (f–n). Add salt and pepper to taste.

7. Pack the mixture into the mason jar (o).

8. Pour the sauerkraut juice over the salsa so that it is covered (p). Use at least 1 cup (235 ml) of the sauerkraut juice, or more as needed to cover up the vegetables. Leave 1 inch (2.5 cm) of headroom.

Pico de Gallo *(continued)*

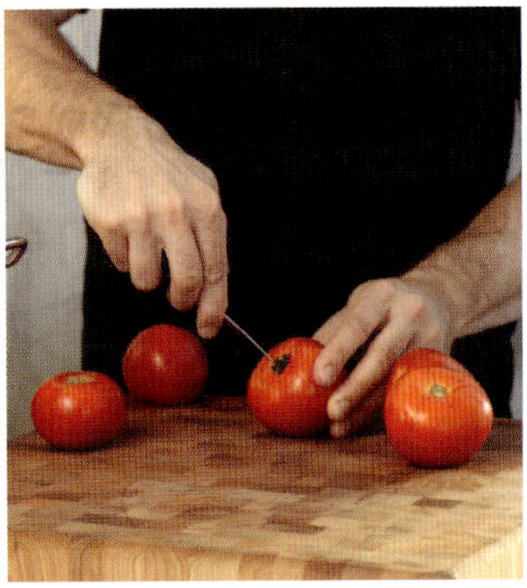

a

9. Close the lid and leave the mixture on the counter for 3 to 5 days. Then transfer it to the refrigerator, where it will keep for at least a couple of weeks, and probably much longer.

Pico de gallo is a versatile condiment and flavoring. Have it with an avocado, with sour cream or crème fraîche, or with cheese. Try it on grilled fish, other grilled foods, or with lighter meats. And, of course, you can eat it with tortilla chips!

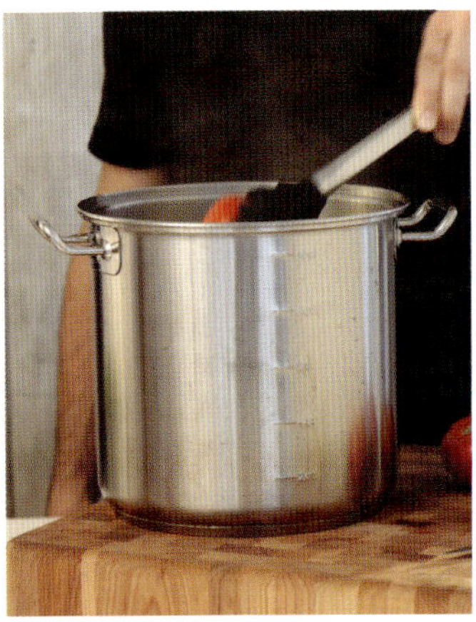

b

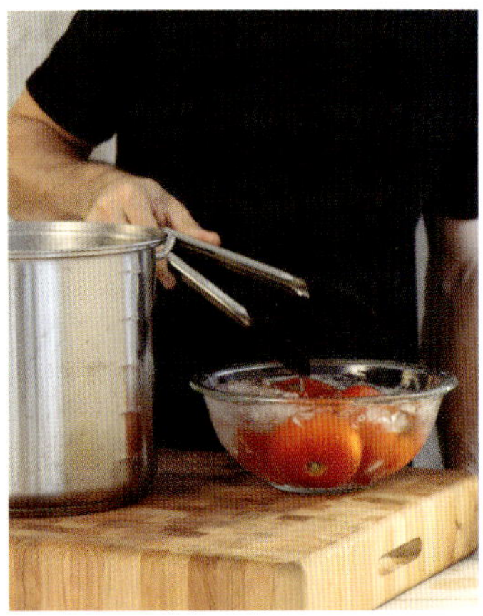

c

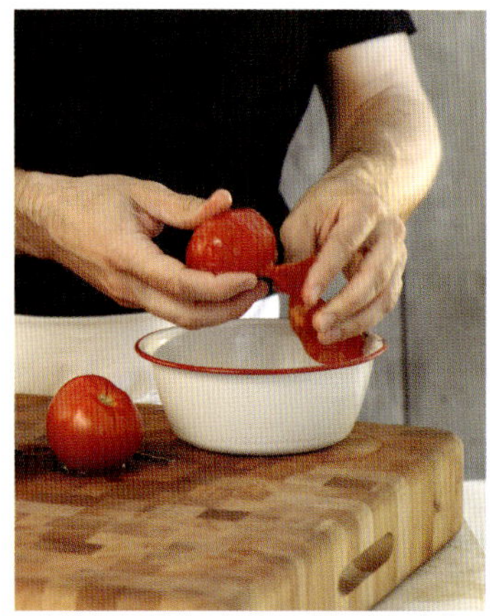

d

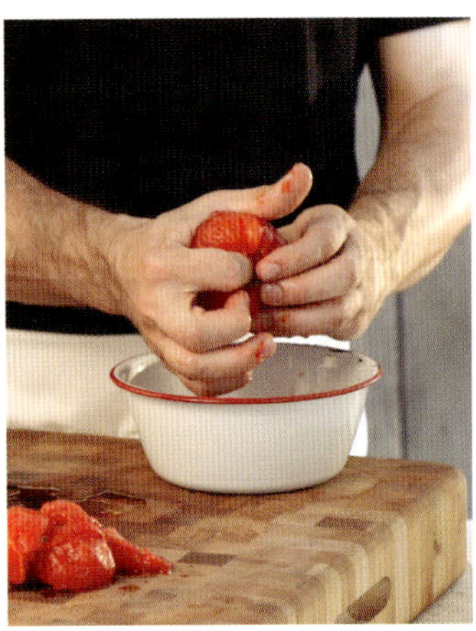

e

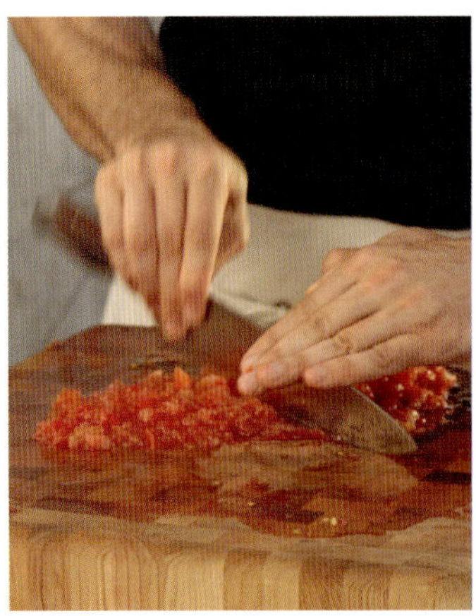

f

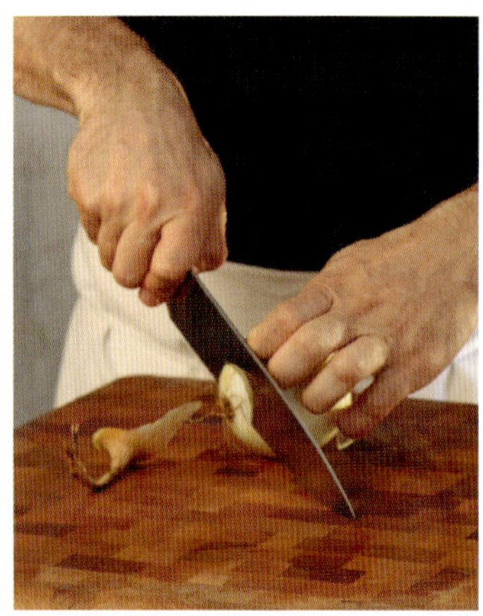

g

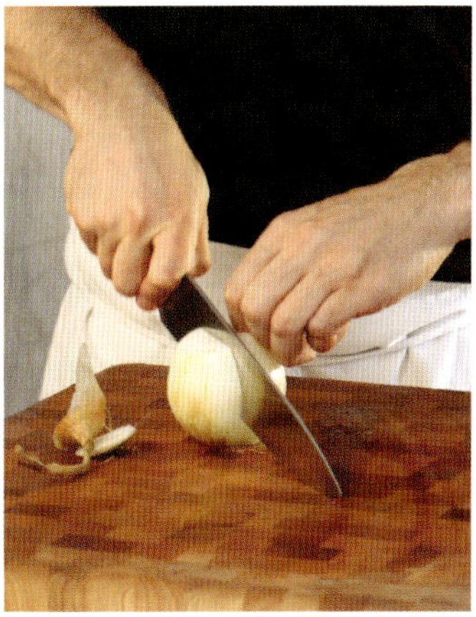

h

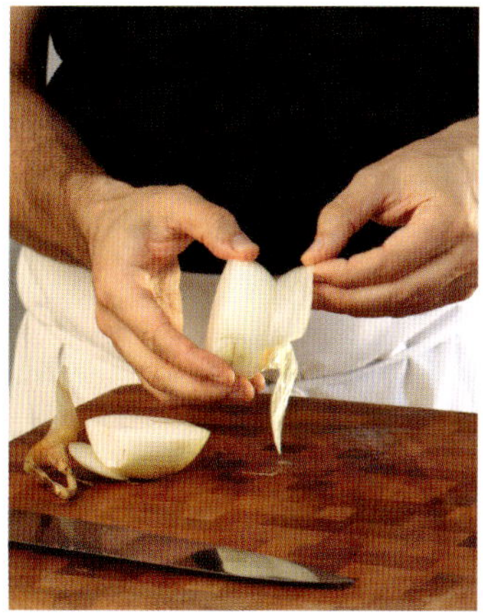

i

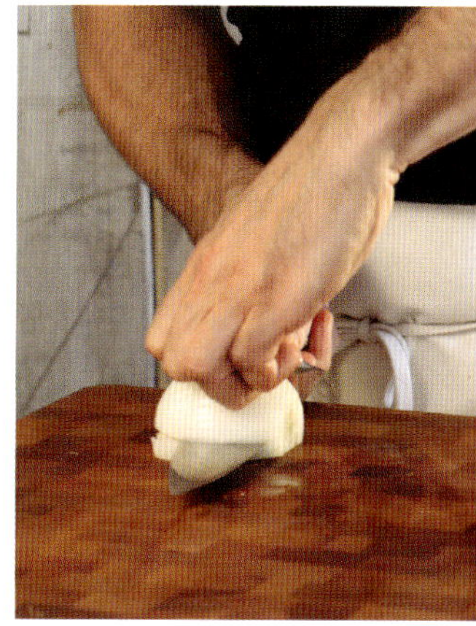

j

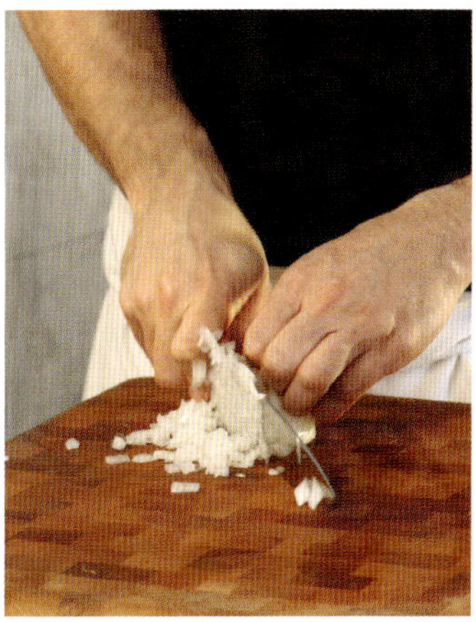

k

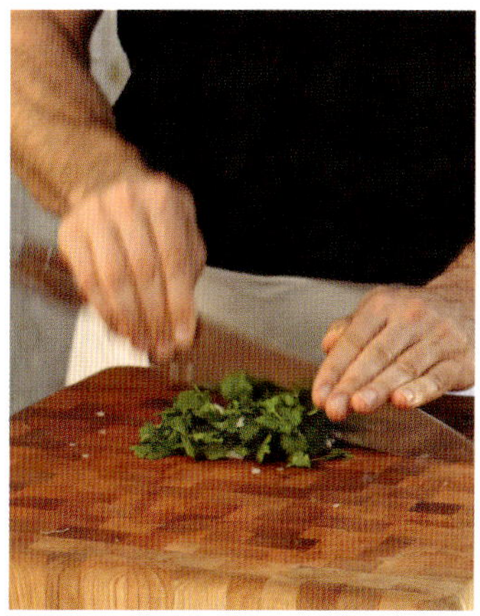

l

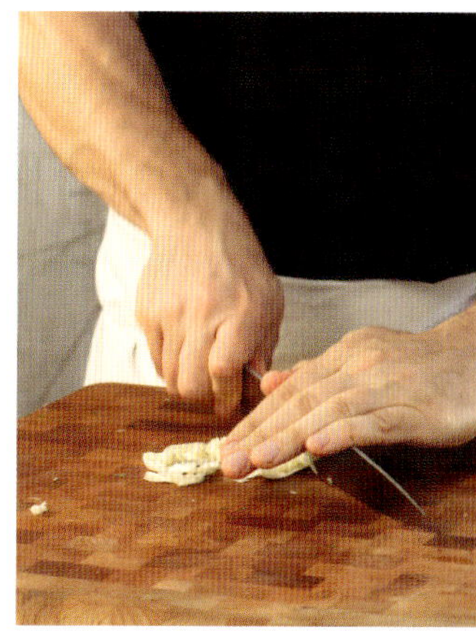

m

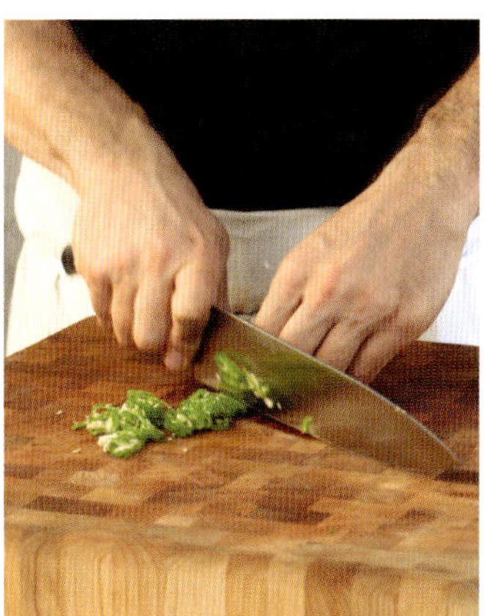

n

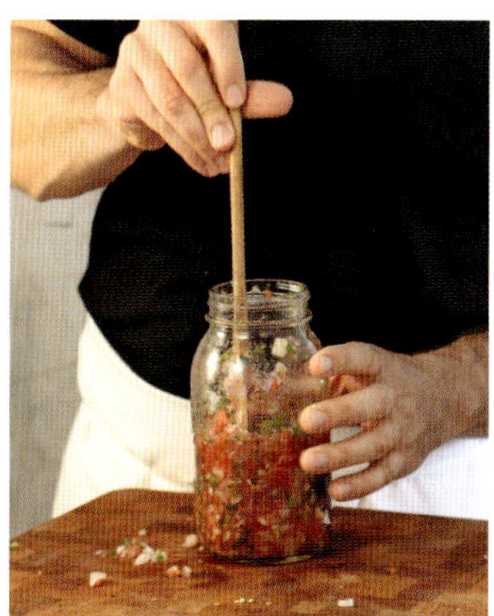

o

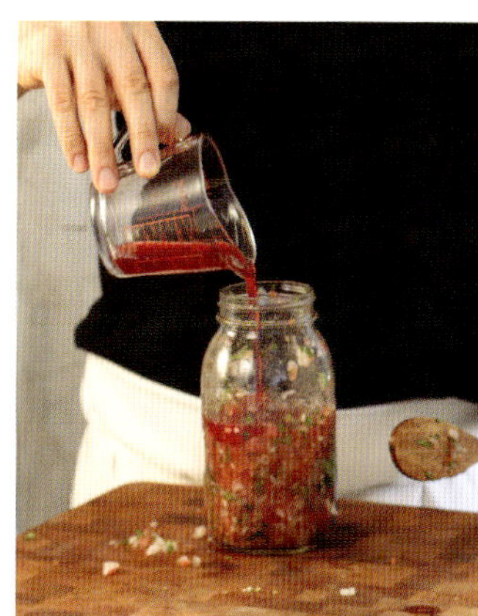

p

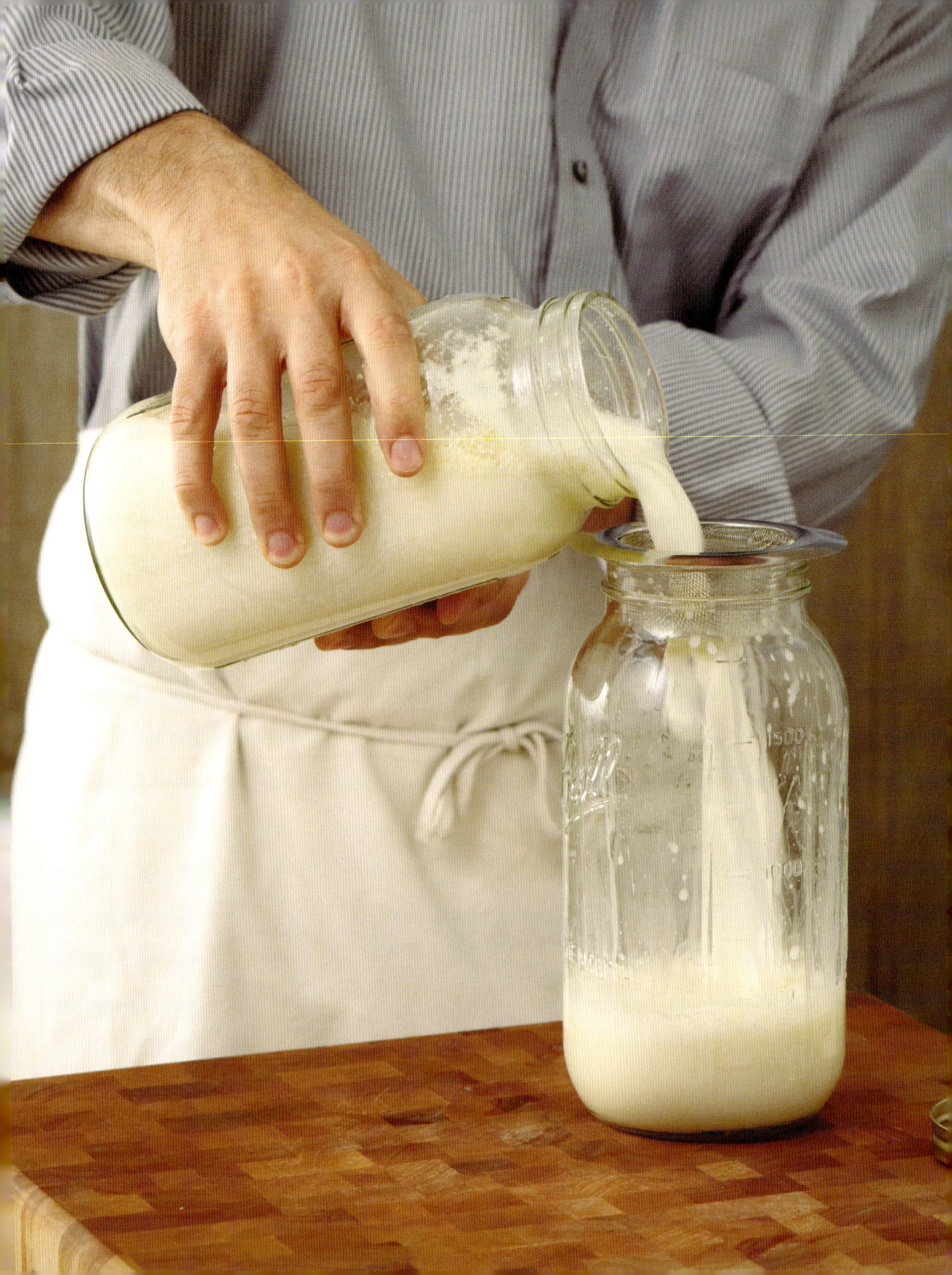

CHAPTER 6

Fermented Beverages

The most popular, interesting, and important beverages in the world are fermented. Before you dismiss this as hyperbole, consider this partial list: coffee, chocolate, and some kinds of tea; every alcoholic beverage, including wine, beer, hard apple cider, mead, sake, and hard liquor; vinegar and kombucha; and dairy beverages based on yogurt and kefir, discussed in chapter 4. All of these are fermented!

Coffee and chocolate are both edible in their raw plant state, but their raw states are quite different from their familiar forms, and in order to effect the transformation, they are processed by various methods, including fermentation. Fermentation is used to transform many different foods into beverages, imbuing them with desired qualities such as acidity, alcohol, or additional flavors. In every case, the creation of these drinks relies on the actions of microbes.

It may not come as a complete surprise that so many important beverages are fermented. Given sufficient time, many beverages will ferment on their own, often with acceptable results. But when we involve ourselves in the process, we can guide it toward a particular goal, further ensuring that the outcome is to our liking.

Kombucha

PREP TIME: 20 MINUTES • TOTAL TIME: 5–15 DAYS

Kombucha, also known as "tea kvass," is a fermented beverage that typically contains very little alcohol, so it is generally considered nonalcoholic. Kombucha is not nearly as universal as wine and beer, and its history is not as well understood. Despite this, or perhaps because of it, kombucha has developed pockets of dedicated followers.

Current and former kombucha fans include characters as diverse as Aleksandr Solzhenitsyn, Ronald Reagan, and Madonna. Kombucha's healing properties have been widely discussed and pondered. Partly because there is not a large global market for kombucha, not as much formal research has been done into its biochemistry. But it contains a variety of bacteria, healthy yeasts, and enzymes, like many other fermented foods, so it has similar benefits. Recent research does suggest that kombucha's glucaric acid may be an effective liver tonic, helping the liver eliminate waste (including waste from chemotherapy), and that kombucha microbes may help the gut maintain a good balance of bacteria.

INGREDIENTS

Approximately 2 quarts (2 L) nonchlorinated water

2 teaspoons (10 g) *plain* black, oolong, or green tea (or a combination), loose or in bags (tea bags are typically 2 to 4 g each)

½ cup (133 g) sugar

¾ cup (175 ml) kombucha starter, from a previous, recent batch

1 piece kombucha "mother" (at least several square inches [20 or more cm2] in area), also known as SCOBY

EQUIPMENT

4-quart (4-L) saucepan with lid

Clean 3-quart (3-L) or larger glass jar or jug (clean it with boiling water)

Clean metal spoon (clean it with boiling water)

continued

PREPARATION

1. Put the water in the saucepan and bring it to a boil. Turn off the heat.

2. Place the tea in a large jar, pour the boiling water over it (a), put the lid on, let the mixture steep for 10 to 15 minutes, and remove the tea (by removing the bags, or by straining if the tea is loose).

3. Add the sugar to the brewed tea (b), and stir with a metal spoon until it is dissolved. Put the lid back on, and let the mixture cool to approximately room temperature.

4. Add half the kombucha starter to the glass jug, and then add the "mother" (c) and the remainder of the starter (d). (The "mother" may float or sink; it's okay either way.)

5. Cover the top of the jug with the handkerchief and rubber band to keep flies and other foreign objects out (e). Carefully move it somewhere that will maintain warm room temperature, away from direct light.

continued

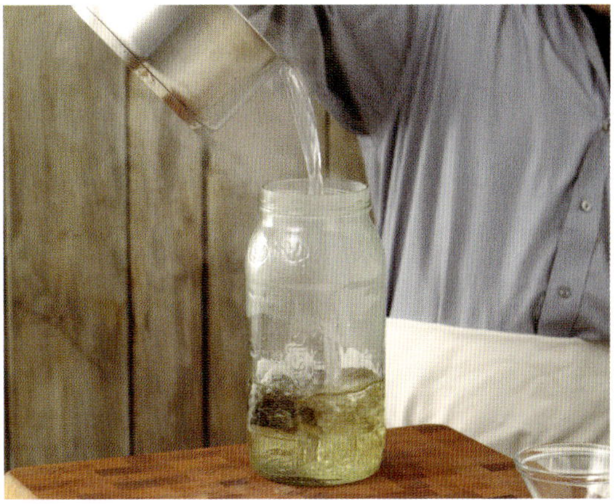

a

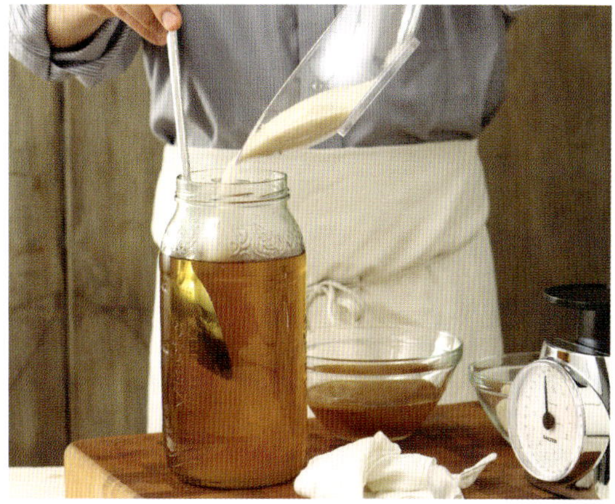

b

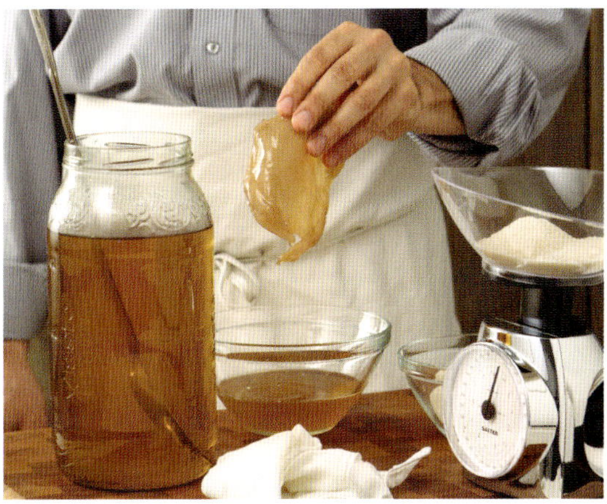

c

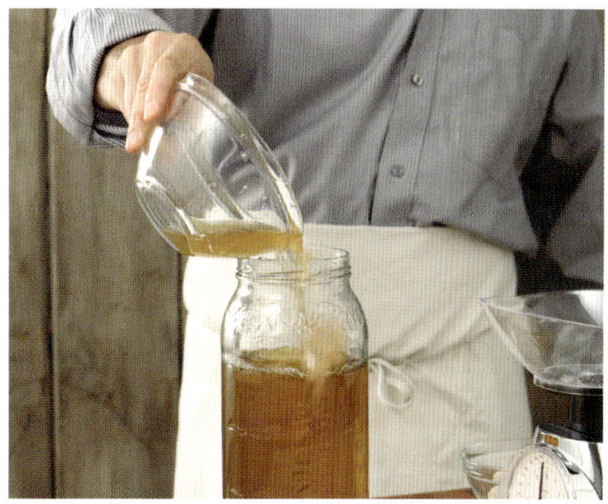

d

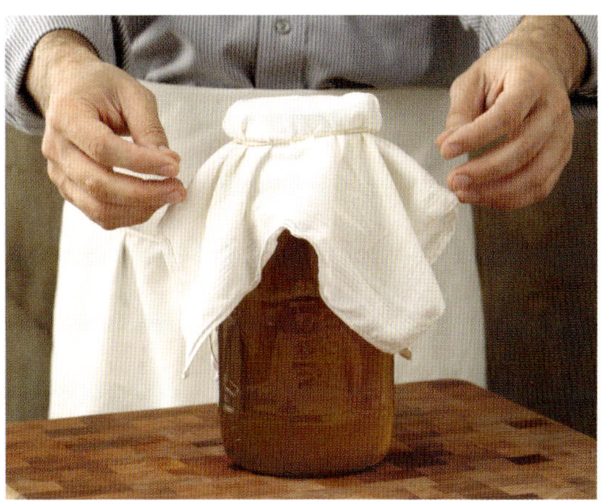

e

Kombucha *(continued)*

Clean white handkerchief or towel and a rubber band that can cover the top of the jug or jar

Large ladle

4 or 5 mason jars (1 pint, or 500 ml each) for storing the finished kombucha

—

Yield: 2 quarts (2 L)

6. After 5 days, start tasting your kombucha with a very clean spoon (you can rinse the spoon in boiling water before using it). The brew should be tart but not unpleasantly sour. If it is still sweet, let it brew for another few days, then taste it again.

7. When you are happy with your kombucha, pour or ladle most of it into mason jars, leaving a bit of room at the top of each. Store them at a cool room temperature or in the refrigerator. Reserve some of the kombucha plus the "mother," and use these to start your next batch.

8. If you like, you can give some of your extra "mother" and some starter to a friend. Wash your hands carefully, pick up the "mother," cut it with a clean knife if necessary, and put it in a jar with some liquid. Keep for yourself at least as much "mother" as you used in your previous batch. If your next batch will be larger, then keep more.

To brew a batch that's bigger than 2 quarts (2 L), scale the recipe accordingly. So for each quart (1 L) of water, you will use ¼ cup (67 g) sugar, 1 teaspoon (5 g) loose tea (or two teabags), and 6 tablespoons (90 ml) starter liquid, plus, of course, your SCOBY.

SCOBY FROM SCRATCH

If you can't find a kombucha SCOBY, but you have access to kombucha in your supermarket, you can try creating a SCOBY by starting from a bottle. Follow the recipe here, use your bottle of kombucha as the starter, and skip the part about the SCOBY. It may take substantially longer than 5 to 15 days, and it might simply not work. It might work, however, and if you find yourself with a SCOBY, you can make more (and more) kombucha for yourself from that one purchase. Your chances will be best if you can find a "traditional" kombucha to start with rather than a "reformulated" one. The traditional kombuchas are often sold as alcoholic beverages because they may contain 0.5 to 1.5 percent alcohol.

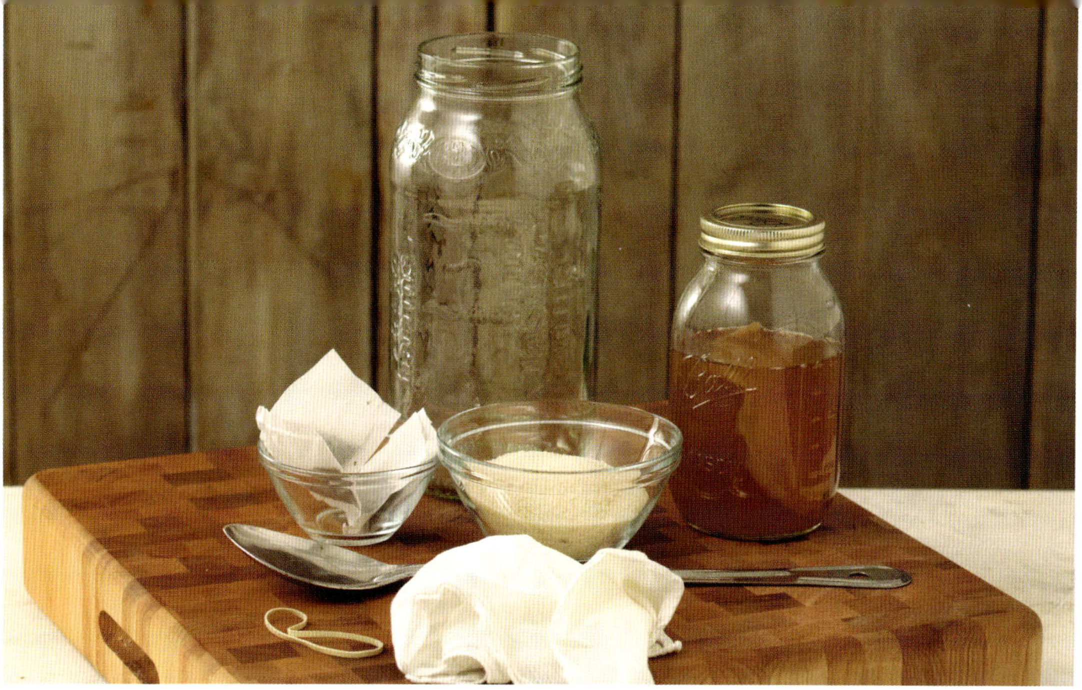

Equipment and ingredients for making kombucha

THE KOMBUCHA MOTHER: SCOBY

The cellulosic mat known as the "mother," "SCOBY," or "tea mushroom" is kombucha's signature trait. In appearance and texture it resembles a flat piece of abalone or squid. SCOBY is an acronym for "Symbiotic Culture of Bacteria and Yeast." This mat is both the by-product of kombucha fermentation and the medium on which the bacteria and yeast live. Sometimes the SCOBY is called a "mushroom"; this is inaccurate. To get started making kombucha, you will want to find a SCOBY and some kombucha liquid. These can be bought over the Internet, but depending on where you live, you may be able to find someone giving them away near you, because every time you make a batch of kombucha, a new SCOBY forms.

Besides the SCOBY, kombucha's ingredients are very simple: water, tea, and sugar. As always, use chlorine-free water. If you boil tap water for 10 or 15 minutes, most of the chlorine will evaporate. For more information about water, see page 34.

Plain, organic black, oolong, or green tea is the best choice. The spices used in flavored teas can sometimes interfere with the bacteria and yeast; for instance, bergamot, used in Earl Grey tea, has antimicrobial properties. Not surprisingly, the preservatives and chemicals used on nonorganic tea can also have antimicrobial properties.

Finally, any kind of sugar is fine to use, although if you are seeking to avoid GMOs (see page 32), you may want to skip beet sugar, which is often GM, and get cane sugar, which is not. And if you would like to get some extra trace minerals, turbinado sugar is excellent. Don't worry about the large amounts of sugar involved in the making of kombucha; most or almost all of the sugar gets metabolized by the SCOBY and converted into acids. For exactly this reason, artificial and/or noncaloric sweeteners will not work; the SCOBY will only eat actual sugar.

The more sour the kombucha, the more sugar that has been converted.

LAB NOTES

If you buy kombucha from the store, you can save the bottles and use them for storing your own homemade kombucha. The jars tend to be 16 ounces (500 ml) and made of thick glass, so they're suitable for this application.

If you don't want to start your next batch immediately, you can store your kombucha starter and "mother" in a jar in the refrigerator for a couple of months.

The longer you store your finished, bottled kombucha at room temperature, the more carbonation you may get.

If you use plain black, oolong, or green tea (or a combination), it is possible to maintain a kombucha SCOBY lineage indefinitely. But if you would like to experiment with using a kombucha starter to ferment herbal teas, flavored teas, barley tea, fruit juice, and so on, feel free. In this case, it is always wise to keep some extra tea-only starter and "mother" on hand and to continue brewing them using plain tea, so that there is a fallback if your experimental strain eventually fails.

Exotically flavored kombuchas are popular and are available in many stores. Strawberry, mango, ginger, blueberry, and spirulina all find their way into kombucha. If you want to make flavored kombucha at home, purée your flavorings and add them to jars of finished kombucha. Store these flavored kombuchas on a shelf for a while before refrigerating, to get carbonation and a more thorough blending of flavors. Adding the flavorings at the end is better than adding them during brewing. Some flavorings attract the wrong sorts of microbes if added too soon; others, like ginger, have antimicrobial properties that could potentially affect fermentation. Note that the sugar in these flavorings may cause additional buildup of carbonation. Open your bottles periodically to make sure you are not heading toward an explosion!

Kombucha Mother: An Owner's Manual

By Annabelle Ho, author of the blog Kombucha Fuel, www.kombuchafuel.com

Every time you brew a batch of kombucha, a new kombucha mother—the SCOBY—typically forms on the surface. Ideally, a healthy kombucha mushroom is a cream-colored, ⅛"–¼"-thick pancake. If your kombucha culture does not fit this description, do not worry! Many factors, such as low and inconsistent brewing temperatures, different brewing environments, brewing duration, and more, can affect the kombucha mushroom.

Younger mushrooms tend to have a light, creamy color, which develops into a darker brown color as the cultures age. An incompletely formed mushroom or a SCOBY with varied thicknesses is perfectly fine to use for most individuals' home-brewing purposes. In addition, because the kombucha mushroom grows on the surface of the container that it ferments in, SCOBYs will always take on the shape of the container.

Younger mushrooms tend to perform (or ferment) better than older ones do. Once you've grown a good, young mushroom, you can store the older one in the refrigerator as a backup or give it to friends.

If you don't see a new mother forming on the surface of your kombucha, here are some tips:

- **Sleeping SCOBY:** Was your SCOBY stored in the fridge? Kombucha mushrooms go "dormant" in the fridge and may need a few cycles to get fully back into gear. Wait a few cycles to see whether new SCOBYs begin forming.
- **Conjoined SCOBY:** Is your kombucha mother sitting on the surface of the kombucha as it brews, and is it getting thicker? If it is, then there's a good chance that the new mushroom is forming right on top of the old one, and the two mushrooms are indistinguishable from each other.
- **Room to breathe:** Be sure to leave a few inches (cm) of air space at the surface of the fermentation vessel to allow room for the baby SCOBY to grow.
- **Shelve the soap:** Avoid cleaning your brewing vessel and equipment with antibacterial soap because SCOBYs contain bacteria. Distilled white vinegar can be used to clean your kombucha equipment and brewing vessel prior to use instead.
- **Caution:** hot. Don't add SCOBYs to hot or warm tea because hot temperatures can kill the culture. Add SCOBYs to sweetened tea that is at room temperature.
- **No smoking!** Avoid brewing in environments where there is smoke (including smoke from cooking), pollen, or toxic fumes such as from paints or solvents.
- **Stay out of the sun:** Do not brew on a windowsill where there is direct sunlight.
- **Stay still:** Keep your fermentation vessel in an undisturbed spot. Every time you move the fermentation vessel while it is brewing, the new baby mushroom begins forming all over again.
- **Keep it simple:** Use only plain, unflavored, and raw kombucha as starter (from the previous batch or purchased from a store). Remember to avoid any foreign additions and flavors when brewing kombucha (such as herbs, spices, certain types of tea, etc.) and to only add these to finished kombucha.

- **Stay sweet:** Ensure that your sweetener contains some form of sugar in either a dry or a crystalline form, such as evaporated cane juice or Sucanat, or in a liquid form, such as honey. Stevia and artificial sweeteners do not provide the necessary food for the yeasts.
- **Age matters:** The ability for SCOBYs to ferment the tea and to produce new babies tends to decrease as they age. Older SCOBYs are darker brown in color while younger SCOBYs typically have a creamy, white color.

Growing a Thick Kombucha Mushroom

Because the kombucha may be ready to drink before a well-formed kombucha mushroom fully develops, growing a nice, thick kombucha mushroom is not always synonymous with brewing delicious kombucha. However, having a thick SCOBY can be advantageous as thicker mushrooms tend to ferment the tea more effectively, to a certain extent. A ⅛"- to ¼"-thick mushroom is healthy.

To grow a thick kombucha mother, you can put some unflavored and raw kombucha in a clean glass jar, cover it with a breathable cloth, and secure the cloth with a rubber band. Let it sit for a few weeks in a warm, undisturbed spot until a thick mother grows and develops. Alternatively, allow one of your kombucha brews to ferment for a prolonged period of time until a thick SCOBY forms. The process may take several weeks.

The kombucha will become strong, sour, and acidic if it has been fermenting for a long time, which you may not want to drink. This tea can be used as starter tea, however.

Brewing Rate

There are two significant factors that can affect the rate of the brewing process:

- **Temperature:** Kombucha brews ideally at around 75°F–85°F (25°C–30°C). Kombucha can brew at temperatures slightly above and below that range. However, if the temperature is lower than mid 60°F (around 18°C), use something to increase the temperature of your brew, such as a seedling mat.
- **The amount of starter tea used:** Typically it is recommended to use around 10 to 20 percent starter tea in the overall brew. During the warmer months, you can use closer to 10 percent of starter tea, because fermentation will be faster. In the colder months, use closer to 20 percent starter tea to help get the fermentation process going.
- **SCOBY Storage:** Refrigerating the Kombucha Mushroom

Refrigerating the kombucha mushroom is usually the easiest method for SCOBY storage between batches. Store the kombucha mushroom in a glass jar with some unflavored kombucha tea. Or, kick-start the brewing process for several days to get the pH level down, and refrigerate the mushroom in its brewing container. This will make the kombucha culture "dormant." It won't be completely inactive, but the SCOBY will be active at a very slow rate, and it can keep this way for months. Keep the lid closed only loosely, so that carbon dioxide doesn't build up and pop the top off.

Consider giving the SCOBY some fresh air and oxygen by opening the lid every now and then. If the kombucha mushroom is in the refrigerator for several weeks or more, it is recommended to add some sweet tea to it every now and then, to give the yeasts additional sugars to feed on. If you would like to resume brewing with a mushroom that has been stored in the refrigerator, allow the SCOBY stored in kombucha to warm up to room temperature overnight before use. When you begin brewing again, it may also take a few cycles for the SCOBY to kick back into full gear.

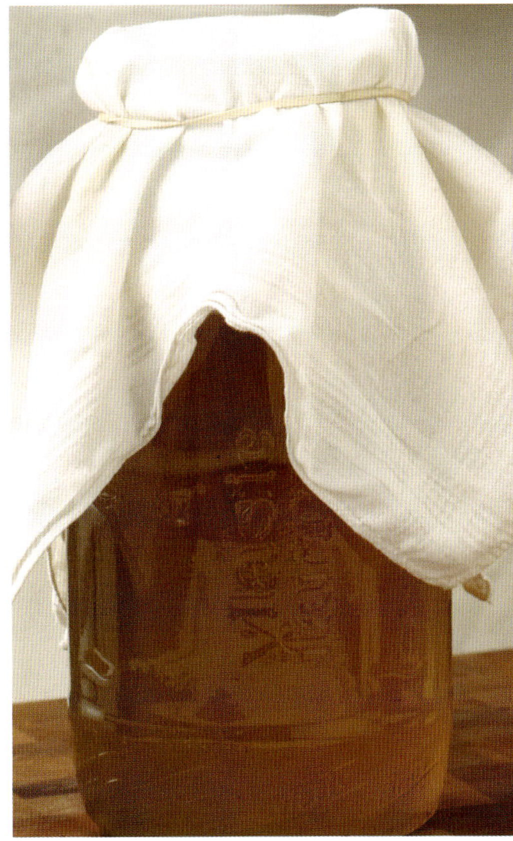

Mold

When kombucha is brewed properly and with good kitchen sanitation, the chance of mold contamination is low, because kombucha's anti-microbial properties and acidic pH protect it. If mold does appear, it will be on the top of the SCOBY, and will look fuzzy, like the mold on food and bread. When this happens, the SCOBY and the batch of kombucha should be thrown out, to be safe.

Vinegar

PREP TIME: MINIMAL • TOTAL TIME: MONTHS; VARIES

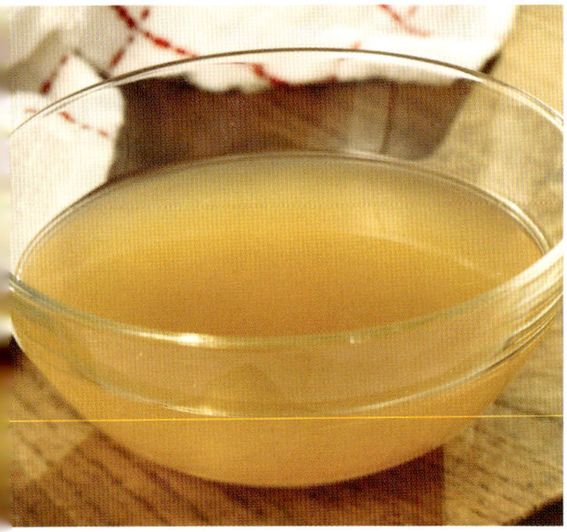

Vinegar is traditionally made by the further fermentation of an alcoholic liquid: bacteria convert the alcohol into acetic acid. These bacteria can either be wild, finding the liquid on their own, or they can be added by us. As vinegar ferments, a sort of floating mat can form. This mat is analogous to the mat that forms during the brewing of kombucha (see page 98), and is similarly called the "mother" or "mother of vinegar." Sometimes this is filtered out of the vinegar before use, and sometimes vinegar is pasteurized prior to sale or distribution to prevent the formation of more mother.

Vinegar is typically not drunk straight. It is sometimes mixed with water and perhaps a sweetener or some herbs—sometimes as a digestive or liver tonic, or for medicinal purposes. Raw vinegars have more tonic properties than pasteurized ones because of the live bacteria, and in fact, an ounce (30 ml) or so of raw apple cider vinegar, diluted with water, is recommended by some as an excellent drink to have first thing in the morning.

Vinegar's widest application these days is as a recipe ingredient. Vinegar has many culinary uses. Because of its high acidity, it is useful and effective for preserving food. It also provides a sharp or sour flavor for dishes that would otherwise lack bite. It is popular with leafy vegetables to offset their sometimes bitter flavor; with meats it was used along with spices before refrigeration to mask rancidity, and where it can also help prevent the palate from being overwhelmed by fat; and with sweet foods.

If you would like to make vinegar at home, wine and hard cider are good starting points. Vinegar, like kombucha, needs some air to ferment; try using an open crock with a cloth over it, stored in a dark place. If you simply add wine or hard cider to a crock and let it stand, you may get good vinegar, but keep in mind that commercially sold wine and cider may contain preservatives, and they may not turn into very good vinegar on their own. Even if it turns into good vinegar, it may take a long time. To help things along, use a starter. You may be able to get a vinegar starter from a friend; otherwise, you can try using some raw apple cider vinegar, which is available in many supermarkets. One part starter in ten or one in twenty should be enough to get things going.

INGREDIENTS
1 quart (1-L) wine, apple cider, or other fermented beverage

¼ cup (60 ml) vinegar from a previous batch, or some store-bought raw apple cider vinegar, to use as starter (optional)

EQUIPMENT
Jar

Handkerchief or towel with which to cover the container; you want to keep foreign matter out but allow the vinegar to breathe

Rubber band or piece of string

—

Yield: 1 quart (1 L), to start

PREPARATION

1. Pour your wine or cider into the vessel.

2. Add the starter, if using—roughly 1 tablespoon (15 ml) for every cup (250 ml) of liquid, or ¼ cup (60 ml) starter per quart (1 L) of liquid.

3. Cover with the cloth, fasten with the rubber band or string, leave in a dark place, and wait. Be patient. Taste the vinegar occasionally to monitor fermentation, but it will likely take one or two months to become fully sour.

Unfinished bottles of wine are great for this recipe. Once you have some vinegar in progress, you can add to it wine from any unfinished bottles that linger in your kitchen.

LAB NOTES

It is important to use a nonreactive vessel for making vinegar. If you are using a crock, be very sure that its glazing is stable and contains no lead.

In most recipes calling for vinegar, you can use incompletely fermented vinegar, somewhere between wine (or cider) and vinegar. A little alcohol in your salad dressing shouldn't be a problem—and if you are going to be cooking your vinegar anyway, whatever residual alcohol there is will likely boil off. But if you or any of your guests are sensitive to alcohol, you may want to stick to commercially produced vinegar, especially if you will be consuming it raw, such as in a salad dressing.

Also, if you are canning, you are better off using commercially produced vinegar. Canning recipes depend on specific levels of acidity in order to be safe. The acidity of commercial vinegar is measured, regulated, and standardized; when you see a bottle of vinegar that is labeled as 5 percent, for instance, this corresponds to a pH level of slightly below 3. When you make vinegar at home, you don't always know how acidic it is. You can buy a kit to measure the acidity of your home-brewed vinegar, but when in doubt use standardized vinegar.

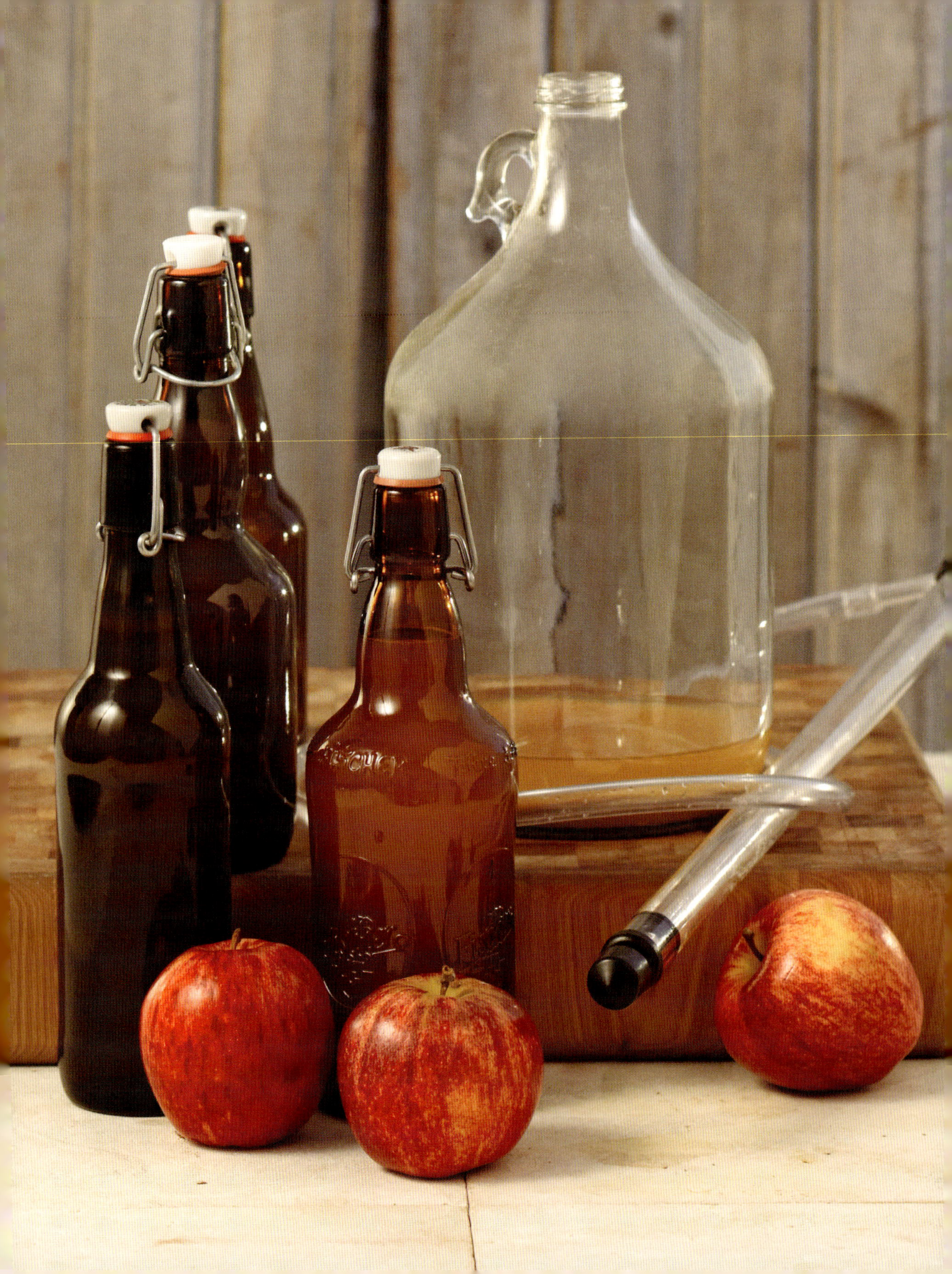

Hard Apple Cider

PREP TIME: 5 MINUTES OR LONGER • TOTAL TIME: 5–15 DAYS

Hard apple cider is one of the easiest alcoholic beverages to make at home.

If you live in an apple-growing region, you might be able to find fresh, unpasteurized apple cider at a farm or a farm stand. (Organic is best, because nonorganic apples are often heavily treated with pesticides.) If you are fortunate enough to have your own apple trees, even better—use juice from your own apples, especially if they aren't great eating apples, which most apples aren't.

If you are able to get unpasteurized apple cider, you may not need this recipe at all. Instead, you can simply let your cider sit, cross your fingers, and within a few weeks, because of natural yeasts, you may have good hard cider, depending on ambient temperatures and other factors.

If you are buying your cider in a store, it has probably been pasteurized. In this case, you will need to use a yeast starter because pasteurization kills the natural yeasts. Using a starter is not a bad thing; it improves the likelihood that your cider will turn out well, and it also gives you a better chance of reproducing your results next time if you come up with a particularly successful cider formula. Even when you start with unpasteurized cider, if you would like to have more control over the process, you can pasteurize your cider yourself, and then ferment it with a starter. In fact, Louis Pasteur's "pasteurization" was originally employed in winemaking.

This recipe is definitely of the "home brew" variety. It is not scientific and will not necessarily make the most sophisticated or refined hard cider, but it is fun and satisfying, provides a good taste of home brewing, and is a good jumping-off point for folks who might go on to do fancier yeast brewing, whether it be cider-, wine-, mead-, or beermaking. The door is open to you.

INGREDIENTS

1 gallon (4 L) fresh, unpasteurized apple cider (or store-bought and home-pasteurized cider)

1 envelope (2 teaspoons, or 8 g) cider yeast, champagne yeast, ale yeast, or wine yeast; or, for a wild starter, 1 cup or so (125 to 150 g) fresh organic raspberries or grapes

EQUIPMENT

6-quart (6-L) or larger stockpot (optional)

Food thermometer (optional)

continued

PREPARATION

1. For a wild starter: If you would like to try using a wild starter, put the raspberries or grapes in a pint mason jar, add a cup (250 ml) or so of cider to cover, close the lid, and leave it somewhere warm. Check on it every day. If, after a few days, the contents of the jar have started to get bubbly, then you have successfully captured a yeast starter from your fruit (a)! If a week goes by and nothing has happened, you can try again, or else buy some yeast.

2. Fill the carboy about three-quarters with fresh cider. (If the cider came in the carboy, then pour yourself a glass and drink it to make some space in the bottle!)

continued

Hard Apple Cider *(continued)*

1-pint (500-ml) mason jar (optional)

1-gallon (4-L) carboy (if you bought the cider in a 1-gallon [4-L] jug, this will do nicely)

Airlock that fits in the top of the carboy (optional)

Beugel bottles, also known as "Grolsch-type" bottles or swing-top bottles (optional)

Auto-siphon pump and some tubing (optional)

—

Yield: 1 gallon (4 L)

3. Add your starter (whether it's a wild starter, as in step 1, or an envelope of yeast) to the carboy of cider (b), cap it, and give the carboy a shake or a swirl.

4. Prepare the airlock, if using, and install it into the top of the carboy. If you are using a simple airlock, as pictured, prepare it by removing the cap, half-filling it with water (up to the line) (c), (d), and then replacing the cap (e).

5. Leave the cider somewhere dark and relatively cool for a couple of weeks.

6. Taste your cider periodically. If you'd like to be scientific, you can estimate the alcohol content of the cider by periodically measuring its specific gravity using a hydrometer. Different hydrometers work in different ways; how you take the measurement depends on the particular hydrometer that you buy. In any case, it is not necessary.

continued

YEAST STARTERS

The most surefire way to get a yeast cider starter is to buy one. Many kinds are available in home-brewing stores and on the Internet. Some are intended specifically for cider, others for beer, and yet others for wine or champagne or mead.

There are many opinions about which packaged yeast is "best" for making cider. Different yeasts, different ambient temperatures, and different fermentation periods will result in different flavors and different alcohol levels. You can play it safe and buy one that is nominally intended for cider, or you can try another kind. You could even try baking yeast, although the results may not be like the hard cider you're used to.

Another way to get a yeast starter is to capture yeast from your surroundings. You might be able to do this by leaving an open glass of apple cider sitting on the counter, but there's a good chance you won't get what you are looking for—mold might win the day, for instance. A better, although still not surefire, way to get a wild starter is from fruit. If you look closely at some organic fruit—raspberries and grapes, for instance—you will see a white powder on the skin. (You can capture these yeasts as described on page 118.) (It is important that the fruit be organic, because nonorganic fruits are routinely treated with antimicrobial agents. This is done partly to prevent yeast from growing on them!)

APPLE CIDER VERSUS APPLE JUICE

Naming conventions vary from place to place, but in North America, the term "apple cider" is used to denote the unfiltered juice of apples, apple juice refers to the filtered juice of apples, and hard apple cider refers to apple cider that has been fermented with yeast and contains alcohol.

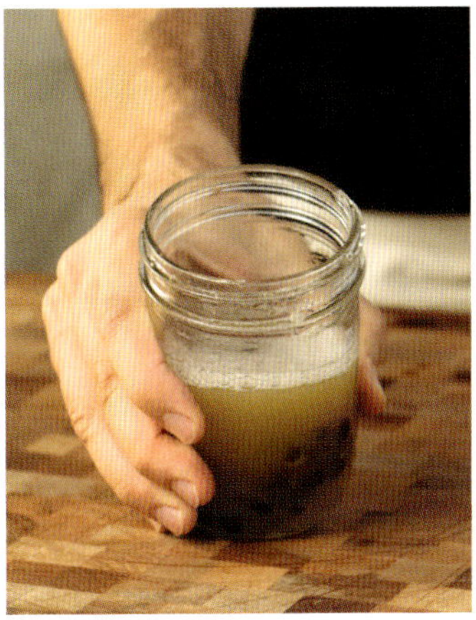

a

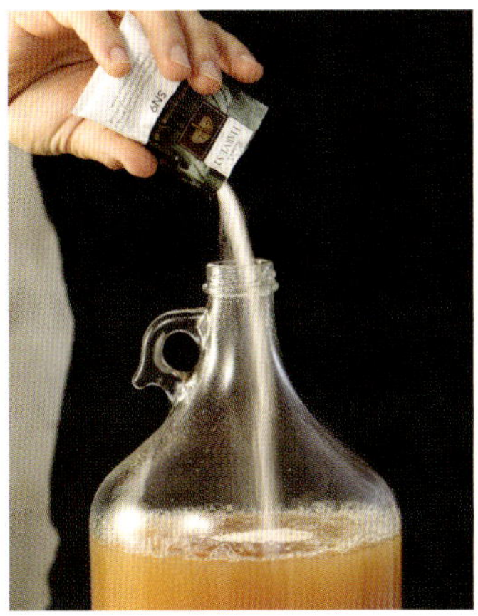

b

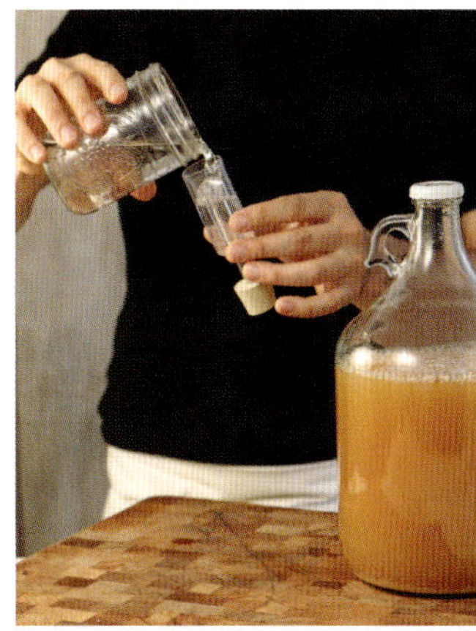

c

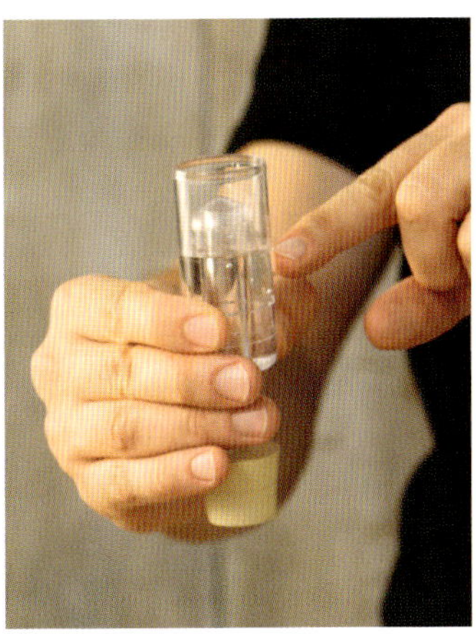

d

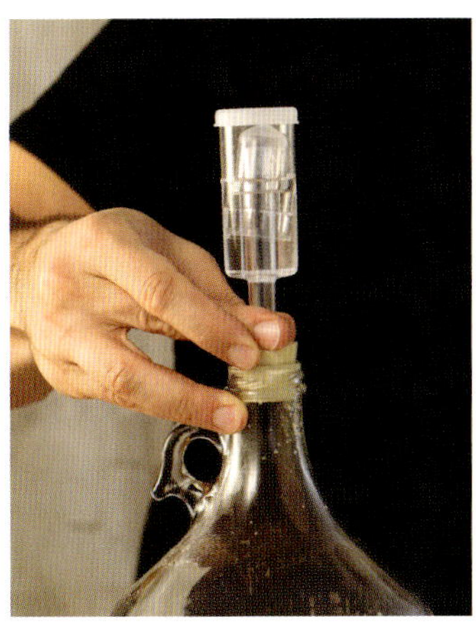

e

Hard Apple Cider *(continued)*

Commercial cidermakers and winemakers use chemicals like sodium metabisulfite to kill the yeasts, thus decisively stopping the fermentation. They do this for reasons of economy, process, and consistency, because it would be too costly and unpredictable for them to have bottles exploding here and there. Sodium metabisulfite and similar chemicals can be toxic if not handled properly, so I do not suggest using them at home, although when added to a cider or wine in proper amounts, they may be safe. Part of the beauty of processing your own food is that you can keep an eye on your cider and release some gas from it if necessary, and you don't have to use chemicals to regularize it.

7. When you are satisfied with the taste, the level of sweetness, and the alcohol content, you can start to drink the cider, and/or transfer it into swing-top bottles, using an auto-siphon if you have one (g), (h). Sediment will probably have settled out of your cider to the bottom of the carboy; if you like your cider clear, then try to avoid disturbing this sediment. (Auto-siphons are designed to avoid disturbing the sediment; they have their inlets some distance above the bottom of the column [i].) On the other hand, if you like cloudy cider, then don't worry about the sediment!

8. If you are moving the cider to bottles, wait until almost all of the sweetness is gone. Too much sweetness means that there is still a substantial amount of sugar left in the cider, which means fermentation will continue in the bottle. If too much fermentation occurs in the sealed bottles, it could result in a buildup of carbon dioxide and, in extreme cases, exploding cider bottles! Swing-top bottles are designed so that the top pops off before the glass breaks, but it is still best to avoid this situation.

9. Leaving the cider to age in the sealed bottles will further mellow its flavor; the aging cider may also gain some fizz. Taste your cider every once in a while. If you are getting a lot of carbonation, you might want to relieve some pressure from the bottles (or they might blow their tops!). Putting your cider in the refrigerator will slow the fermentation significantly.

There's no strict rule for how long you can keep cider, just as there's no strict rule for how long you can keep wine. It might be good after a month, or it might be good after years. The only thing I do recommend is that you open a bottle and taste it periodically; when you think it can't get any better, drink the rest! If it starts to taste too sour, you can keep it around for cooking: as a marinade, use it in place of vinegar in recipes, or even open the tops and see if it will turn into a nice vinegar (see 106).

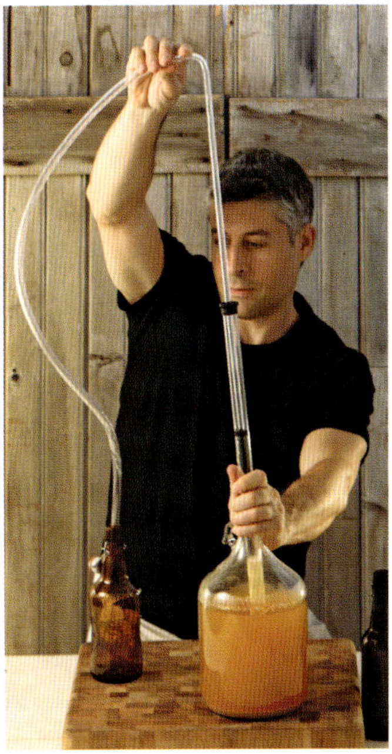

g

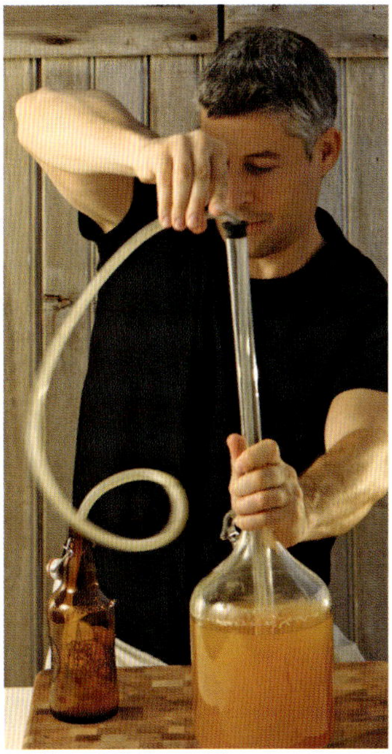

h

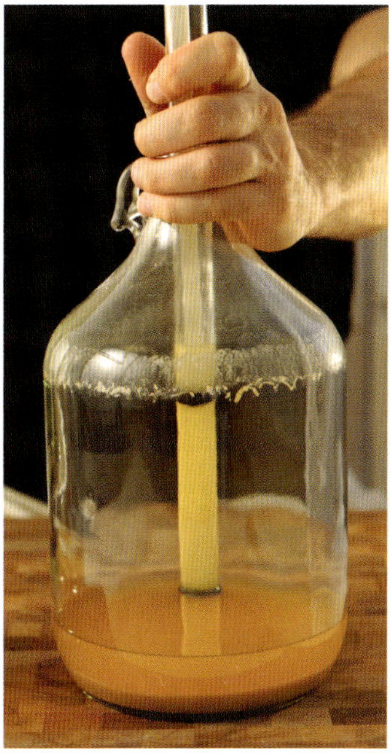

i

LAB NOTES

You can use almost any kind of fruit juice (or carrot juice, or any sweet beverage) as a substitute for apple cider in this recipe. This recipe is a basic template for all yeast-fermented beverages, including wine and beer. So please feel free to experiment with other store-bought juices.

Pear or plum juice will result in something not too far off from the apple version; pomegranate juice will give you something quite different. Give it a try with your favorite juice.

Your results will depend on the sugar content and flavor of the original liquid and the type of yeast you use.

And again, if you are going to store it in closed bottles, it is best to wait until most of the sweetness is gone, to avoid excessive buildup of carbon dioxide that might lead to popped tops.

Mead

PREP TIME: 5 MINUTES OR LONGER • TOTAL TIME: 5–30 DAYS

Mead, also known as honey wine, is a fermented beverage made from honey. Pure honey does not invite microbial activity, but when you dilute it with water—two or three parts water to one part honey—the mixture ferments readily into mead.

Mead is one of the most ancient fermented foods. There are some who theorize that it predates grape wine. It has been an important drink in Asia, Europe, and Africa.

As a home brewer, you can prepare mead in much the same way as you prepare cider. Hybrid fermented beverages are also possible: If you ferment a mixture of honey, water, and apple cider, the result is called *cyser* (see Lab Notes, page 115). You can also ferment a mixture of honey, water, and fruit to get a fruit mead.

INGREDIENTS

2 to 2½ quarts (2 to 2.5 L) nonchlorinated water

1 quart (1.5 kg) honey

1 envelope (2 teaspoons, or 8 g) champagne yeast, ale yeast, or wine yeast; or, for a wild fruit starter, 1 cup or so (125 to 150 g) fresh organic raspberries or grapes

EQUIPMENT

6-quart (6-L) or larger stockpot

Metal spoon

Food thermometer

1-gallon (4-L) carboy (an empty 1-gallon (4-L) apple cider bottle will do nicely)

Airlock that fits into the top of the carboy

Beugel bottles, "Grolsch-type" bottles, or swing-top bottles (optional)

—

Yield: 3–3½ quarts (3–3.5 L)

PREPARATION

1. Put the water into the stockpot and bring it to a boil.

2. Remove from the heat, then add the honey and stir with a metal spoon until well mixed.

3. You have three choices for a starter:

- Use an envelope of yeast.
- Make a wild starter with fruit, as in the Hard Apple Cider recipe (step 1 on page 109), but instead of using apple cider use the honey-water mixture.
- Make a wild starter as in the Hard Apple Cider recipe, but use the honey-water mixture alone, and no fruit.

4. If a significant amount of time has gone by since you combined the water and honey, bring it to a boil again. Regardless, ensure that it is below approximately 100°F (40°C) before proceeding to the next step.

5. Add the starter to the honey-water, stir well, and then pour the mixture into the carboy. Prepare the airlock (as in the Hard Apple Cider recipe, step 4), and insert it into the carboy.

6. Leave the developing mead somewhere dark for a couple weeks. Proceed as for Hard Apple Cider, from step 6.

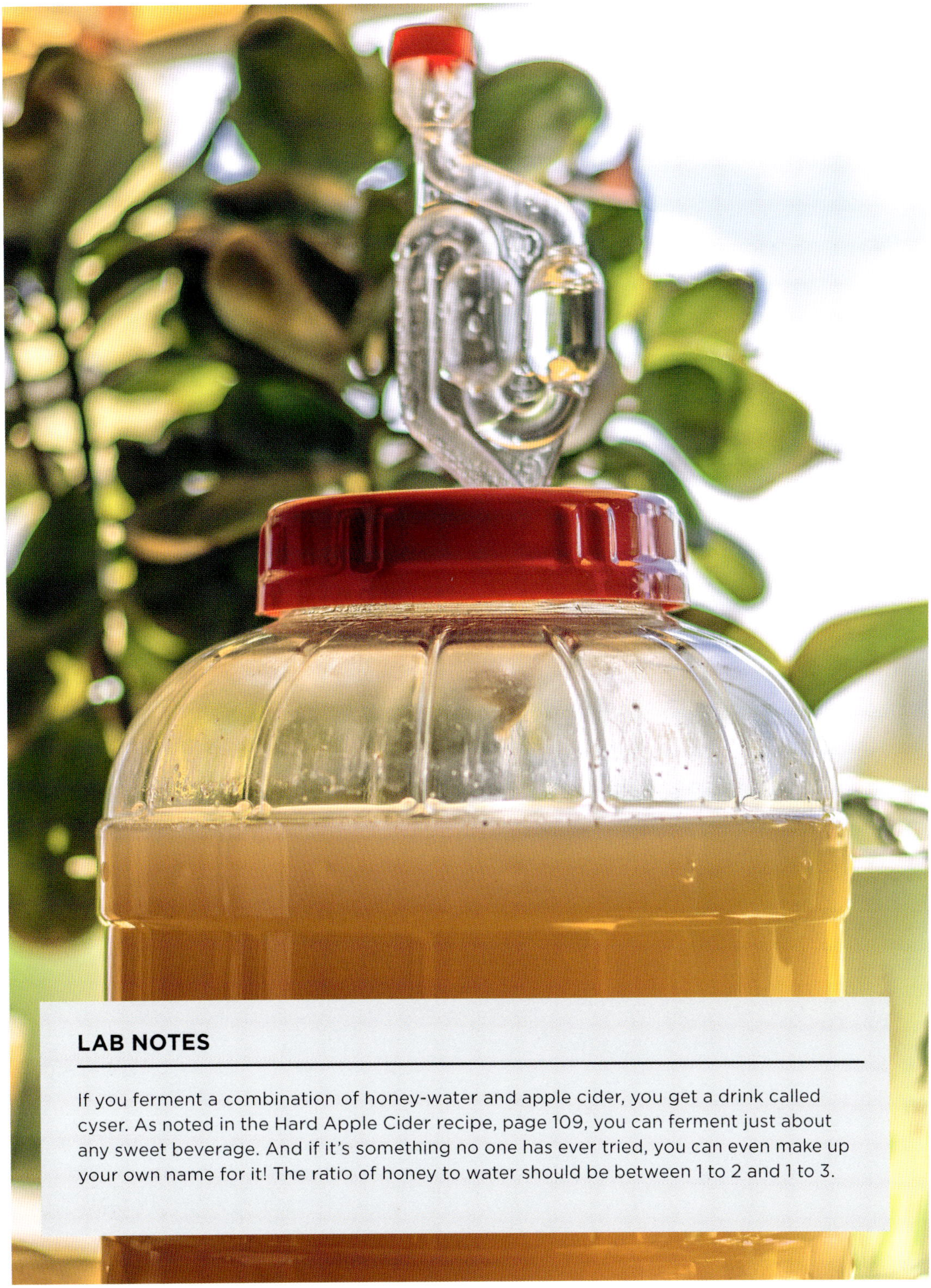

LAB NOTES

If you ferment a combination of honey-water and apple cider, you get a drink called cyser. As noted in the Hard Apple Cider recipe, page 109, you can ferment just about any sweet beverage. And if it's something no one has ever tried, you can even make up your own name for it! The ratio of honey to water should be between 1 to 2 and 1 to 3.

Wine (in Brief)

Wine is one of the most popular and well-known alcoholic beverages in the world. People have been drinking it for thousands of years. It is the result of yeast fermentation of crushed grapes or grape juice, which converts sugars into alcohol, sometimes followed by controlled bacterial fermentation, which changes the acid profile.

There are a lot of subtleties to making good wine. For instance:

- using particular single varieties of grapes, or a specific blend of different varieties (varietals versus blends);
- separating the skins, meat, and pulp from the juice, or leaving them all together for varying lengths of time (this is part of what accounts for different-colored wines);
- adding particular yeasts (most professionally produced wine is made from very specific yeasts);
- aging wines in barrels made of different materials such as oak, stainless steel, or glass, or in bottles;
- using various additives and filtering agents, to help clarify or preserve the wine;
- blending wines from different batches or years before bottling.

Each of these affects the flavor of the wine, its alcohol level, and how it ages.

When the term *wine* is used on its own, it is understood to mean wine made from grapes. Other fruits and fruit juices can also be used to make fruit wines. "Apple wine" and "hard cider" are more or less synonymous, although one or the other term may be preferred, depending on region.

LAB NOTES

If you want to try making wine yourself, you can start by following the basic Hard Apple Cider recipe on page 109; substitute grape juice for the apple cider. The resulting wine may be okay, but it will likely lack the subtlety and refinement of even a modest bottle of professionally made wine.

If you would like to explore further, there are many resources on the Internet that provide ample information about winemaking, and there are entire books dedicated to winemaking. It is a craft that many spend their lives perfecting.

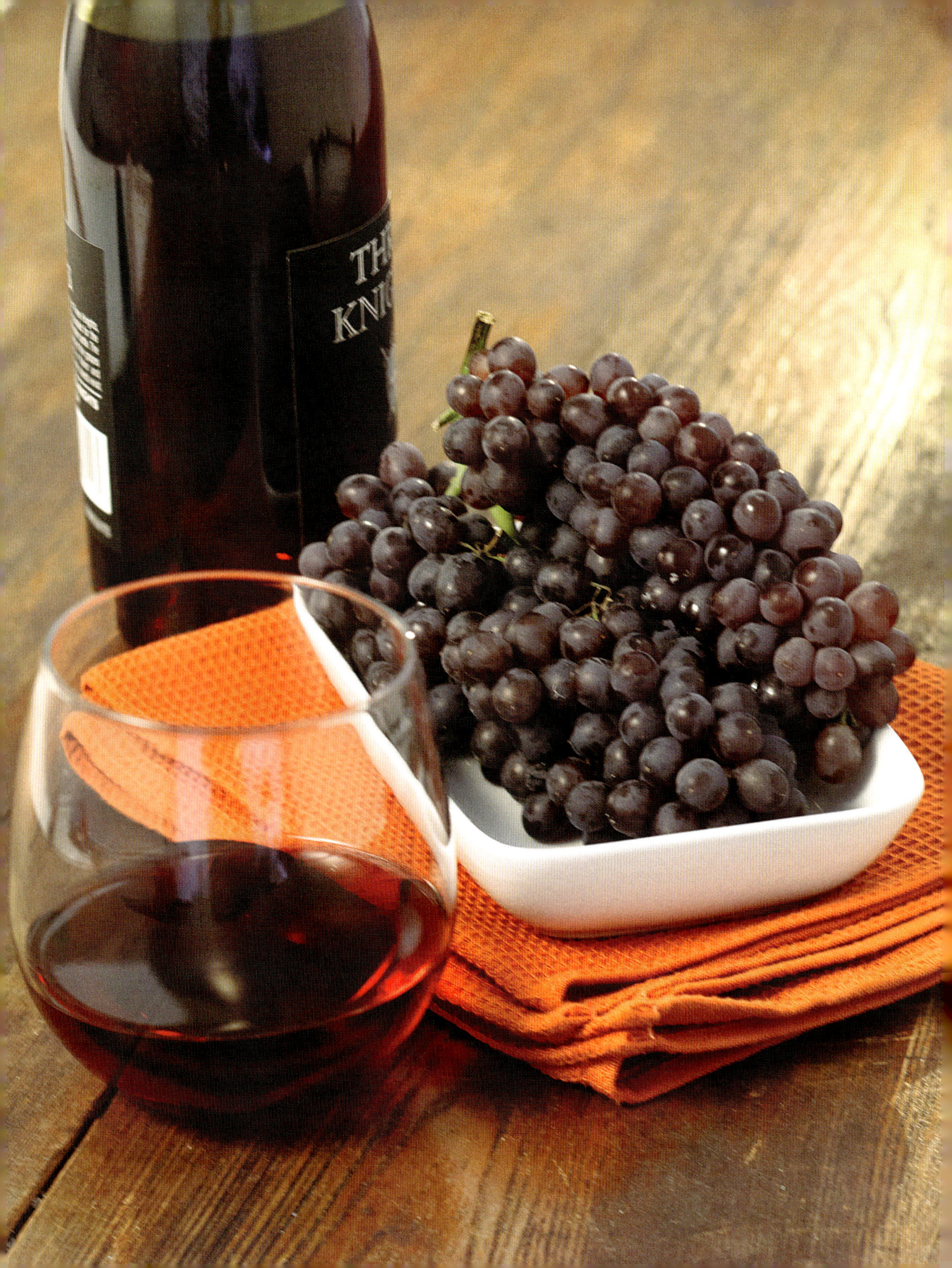

WINE AND FERMENTATION

Corey Beck, general manager and director of wine-making at Francis Coppola Winery in Geyserville, California, gives us a short overview of winemaking.

Put simply, fermentation is the conversion of sugar into alcohol by yeast. Of course, there's much more to the art of making wine than simply adding a bunch of yeast to grape juice. Wine-making starts in the vineyard. Location, weather, soils, rootstock, and clonal selection are all part of winemaking. Once a location is chosen, it takes up to four years before the first grapes will be harvested for wine production. Typically, grapes will be harvested around the 24 to 26 percent sugar range, yielding approximately 14 percent-alcohol wine.

The fermentation process can vary widely depending on the varietal. White grapes are typically loaded directly into a press that squeezes all the juice out of the berries. The juice is then transferred to a stainless steel tank where it will settle for up to 48 hours. The settling process allows for the heavy solids to fall to the bottom of the tank and be removed before fermentation commences. Once the juice has had enough time to settle, the clear juice is racked (transferred) to another tank, and it's there that fermentation begins.

The beauty of fermentation is that there are so many different yeast strains to choose from, each giving the wine unique characteristics. The temperature of the juice when the yeast is added is extremely important. Yeast do not like it when it's too cold; below 50°F (10°C) isn't ideal for them. Most white wines are fermented around 55°F to 60°F (13°C to 16°C); it is at this temperature where most of the wine aromas are being produced from the yeast. Typically, white wine will drop 1 to 2 Brix per day during fermentation, and thus if we start from grape juice with a 24 Brix level, it will take about two weeks for all the sugar to convert into alcohol. (Brix is a measure of the sweetness of a liquid.)

The primary food source in the wine is sugar, and the second is nitrogen, which occurs naturally in grapes. The yeast use these food sources to create three things: heat, carbon dioxide, and alcohol. There are other possible by-products of fermentation; one of them that occurs with Chardonnay grapes is diacetyl, which is the buttery or butterscotch notes in wine. Barrel-fermented wines start off in a tank and then are transferred to barrels to complete the fermentation process. Barrel fermentation gives the wine a richness and vanilla quality that comes from the oak barrels.

Red wine production is somewhat different because the fermentation takes place on the skins of the grapes. Red grapes have clear juice, and the color comes from the pigment in the skins. The grapes are crushed, and the juice and skins are combined in a tank together. Once everything is safely in the tank, yeast are added and fermentation begins. Unlike white wine fermentation, red wine production does best at warmer temperatures, closer to 80°F (30°C). The higher temperatures help extract the color from the red grape skins. Because the temperatures are higher, the yeast are more active and the Brix drop is 4 to 5 per day, so fermentation can be complete in seven days or so. Another compound being extracted from the skins during the fermentation is tannin, which is the flavor building block for red wines. Tannin is what you feel in the sides of your mouth after you drink a Cabernet Sauvignon. Varietals such as Pinot Noir have less tannin, and thus are softer and more approachable at an earlier age. Cabernet Sauvignon has some of the most tannin out of all varietals, and thus takes longer to open up, but will age for years.

Once the fermentation is complete, the pomace is transferred to a press where the remaining juice is squeezed out of the skins. Once the skins have been squeezed they are disposed of and used for compost or fertilizer that goes back to the vineyard. The wine pressed from the red skins will then be transferred to barrels for aging.

Ginger Ale

PREP TIME: 30 MINUTES • TOTAL TIME: 3–7 DAYS

It is easy to make fermented versions of drinks like root beer and ginger ale, or to invent your own fermented soft drinks, at home. The ingredients are simple: water, extracts, and flavorings of your choice, sugar, and a starter. Generally, you can make a fermented soda using any kind of herbal extract or tea as a base. Ginger ale is a good place to start. (For root beer, see "Root Variations," page 121.)

INGREDIENTS

3 to 4 inches (7.5 to 10 cm) ginger root

1 gallon (4 L) nonchlorinated water

1½ cups (300 g) sugar

½ to 1 cup (125 to 250 ml) yogurt whey (see 74), as starter

EQUIPMENT

Box grater or rasp

Stockpot

Large spoon

Carboy with either a tight-fitting cap or an airlock

Several smaller bottles or jars: swing-top bottles, old kombucha bottles, old glass soda bottles, or 1-pint (500-ml) mason jars

—

Yield: 1 gallon (4 L)

PREPARATION

1. Peel and grate the ginger. The edge of a spoon is an excellent instrument for peeling ginger.

2. Add the ginger and the water to the stockpot and bring to a boil. Continue to boil for a couple of minutes. You now have ginger "tea." (It is not tea in the technical sense, because it is not made from the tea plant *Camellia sinensis*.)

3. Remove from the heat, add the sugar, and stir until dissolved.

4. Allow to cool to warm room temperature.

5. Add the whey starter to the sweetened tea.

6. Pour the mixture into the carboy.

7. Prepare the airlock, and install it in the carboy. (If you are not using an airlock, put the cap on, and then open it to "burp" the carboy at least a couple of times a day for the first few days.)

8. Keep the carboy somewhere at room temperature, or a little cooler, for a few days.

9. Your ginger ale should get fizzy in a few days. After a few more days, when the fizz is subsiding, it may be time to bottle it. Pour it into your smaller bottles or jars, and fill them almost to the top, leaving only a little room. Leave these bottles out at room temperature for a few more days, then put them somewhere cool or in the refrigerator.

continued

LAB NOTES

The trick is to bottle your ginger ale while it is still actively fermenting, so that you will trap some carbonation in your bottles—but not so soon that you get too much carbonation for your bottles to contain!

Timing varies greatly, depending on the ambient temperature, but also depending on the activity level of your whey, which is hard to predict. Be prepared for your ginger ale to behave differently every time.

Whey is the easiest starter to use. Anything else that would work for making lacto-fermented sauerkraut (Basic Sauerkraut, page 39) would also work here, although depending on what kind of soft drink you are making, sauerkraut juice may not be the tastiest choice of starter. If you do use sauerkraut juice, be aware that it is not as powerful a starter as whey, so you will need to use more—closer to 1 cup (250 ml) of juice per gallon (4 L) of water.

You can add other seasonings to your ginger ale, including salt, lemon juice, or even fruit juice. Play around with the proportions to suit your taste. You can cut open a vanilla pod, add it to the water, and boil it with the ginger. Most other seasonings and flavorings should be added at the beginning. If you are adding vanilla extract, however, add it at the end.

OTHER CULTURED BEVERAGES

The ancestors of modern sodas were naturally fermented drinks. These traditional beverages typically used decoctions or infusions of medicinal roots, leaves, nuts, or barks as their base, possibly with the addition of some fruit and perhaps a stimulant. Their origins are evident if you look closely at the names of the drinks: "root beer," "ginger ale," "coca," and "cola." They would have been fermented through the addition of sugar and bacterial starter culture, resulting in a slightly sweet, slightly sour, low- or no-alcohol drink containing trace minerals and beneficial bacteria.

The carbon dioxide and phosphoric acid added to today's sodas are meant to evoke the carbonation and acidity that are the natural by-products of fermentation in traditional fermented drinks. Unfortunately, modern sodas have none of the health benefits of traditional fermented drinks, contain far more sugar, and also contain colorings and additives that can be toxic. Consumption of phosphoric acid, for instance, has been shown to lower bone density and cause kidney problems.

Time to Experiment

You are now equipped to perform several different kinds of fermentation on whatever (sweet) liquid you choose, using a variety of starters:

- yeast
- whey
- juice from fermented vegetables
- kombucha starter
- water kefir starter

As an experiment, why not gather a bunch of mason jars, choose a handful of juices or sweet liquids, and try each of a few different starters in each of the different liquids, to see how they all come out? Some will be better than others, and some might not be very good; some will take longer than others, and some might not really work at all. But there is no need to worry about "failure," because this is an experiment. Who knows—maybe you will discover your new favorite drink!

ROOT VARIATIONS

Sassafras, licorice, burdock, dandelion, sarsaparilla, and wintergreen are some of the roots traditionally used for making "root beer." You can experiment with adding these to a ginger ale and reducing the amount of ginger while keeping the ratio of water to sugar the same. Licorice and dandelion are frequently available as herbal teas; burdock is generally easy to find at Asian markets. Sassafras can be found in the wild or bought on the Internet.

Note that some components of sassafras have been found to be carcinogenic to laboratory animals in high concentrations; for this reason, and perhaps because sassafras extract is a precursor to some hallucinogenic drugs, the FDA has banned certain sassafras preparations. But unless you plan on drinking gallons of strong sassafras tea per day, sassafras is probably the least of your worries. For instance, all of the following are probably bigger concerns: eating fried foods (in which carcinogens are formed during the frying process), eating bananas (which are mildly radioactive), or living at high altitudes or traveling on airplanes (where you are exposed to increased levels of radiation due to less atmospheric protection).

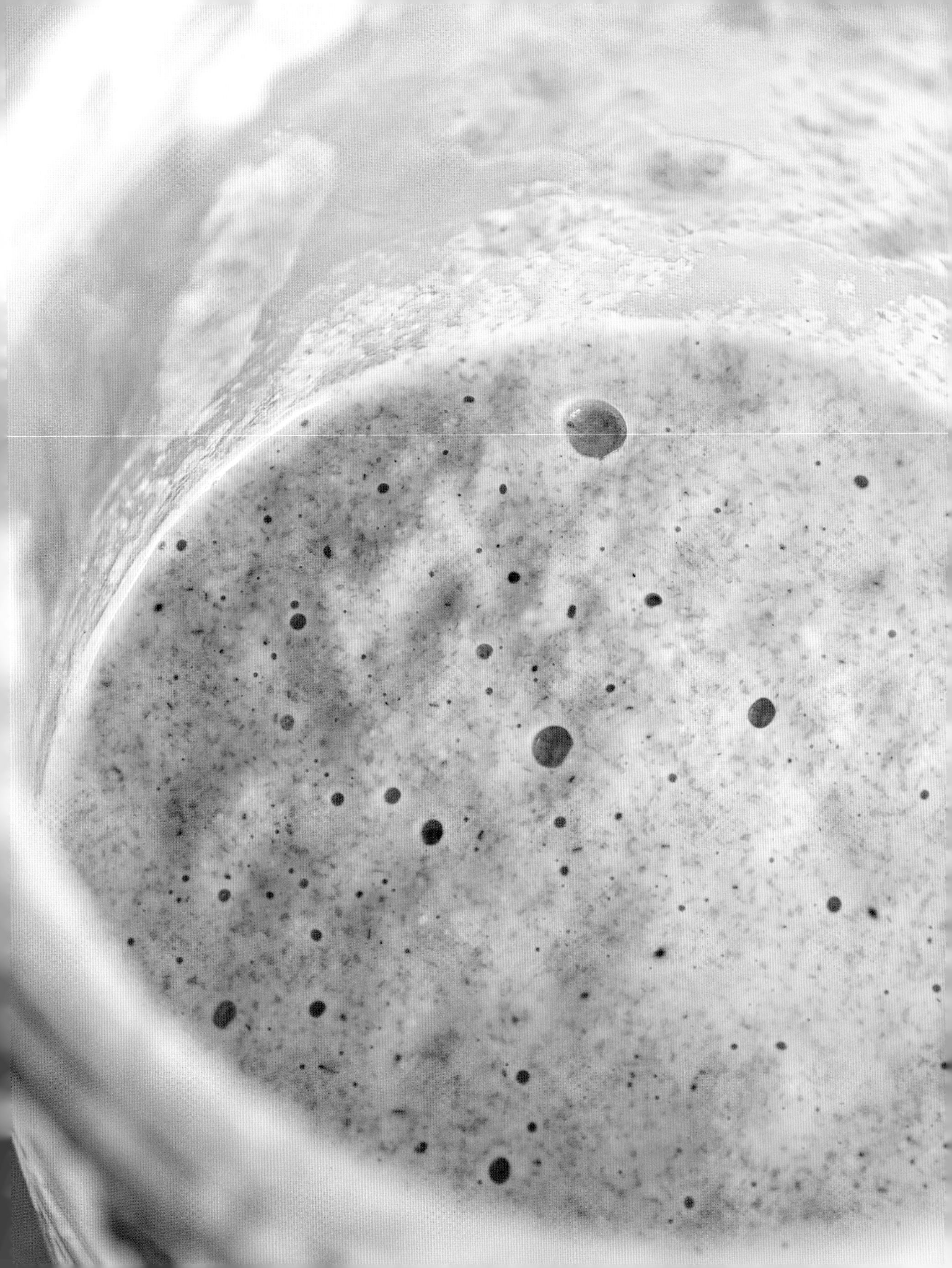

CHAPTER 7

Sourdough

Most modern bread is leavened with dry or fresh yeast, generally manufactured on a large scale. Sourdough bread is leavened with a wild yeast starter that can be saved from a previous sourdough project or if necessary can be pulled from the air. A starter can be perpetuated at any desired scale for months, years, or even centuries.

In this chapter, you'll learn how to capture this wild yeast and how to keep it around in the form of a starter. The starter constantly feeds and grows, so it's good to find things to make with it if you don't make bread all the time. I'll show you a few things I do with this "extra" starter.

A NOTE ABOUT GLUTEN SENSITIVITY

Many gluten-sensitive people are able to eat sourdough bread even when made with flours containing gluten. This is because of the particular ways in which sourdough breaks down gluten proteins. But if you need your foods to be 100 percent gluten-free, then you'll need to use some sort of gluten-free flour or flour mix. Because gluten plays an important role in the texture and structure of bread, gluten-free breadmaking is quite different. If your goal is to make great gluten-free bread, you should seek resources devoted specifically to that topic.

Why Make Sourdough?

I started keeping a sourdough starter for the same reasons most people do: to make bread. But I found that I wasn't always interested in making bread—certainly not more than once a week. In the meantime, as you'll see below, I had to keep the sourdough going, and this meant that I had to find something to do with all the extra starter. (I do my best to avoid throwing away food, not only because it's wasteful but also because it shows a lack of resourcefulness.) The presence of the extra starter led to the porridge and cracker recipes below. Often I found myself more focused on the porridge and crackers and other "discard" recipes than I was on making bread! People come to sourdough to make bread, but in my case, I stayed for other reasons.

As for the sourdough bread itself, part of the appeal is the flavor. Sourdough bread has a pleasingly sour taste and smell. Many people like this. We could speculate about why humans have evolved to enjoy sour things—maybe the taste for sour helps us get adequate vitamin C and avoid acute deficiency, and maybe it encourages us to eat lacto-fermented foods that improve our health and our reproductive fitness in some other way. Conveniently, the higher acidity of sourdough bread also gives it a longer shelf life than a similar bread made with packaged yeast.

A NOTE ABOUT MEASUREMENTS

In most of this book, measurements have been given in Imperial (English) units, with metric equivalents in parentheses. For this chapter only, metric units are given first. Here's why:

The density of dry ingredients can vary. Cups of flour from different sources may weigh different amounts. Banging the cup on the counter may pack the flour more densely. So volume is not a very good way of measuring flour.

Imperial-unit baking recipes typically use volume. But weight is more precise and consistent. And metric weight (grams) is better for math than Imperial weight. (For example, what's 2 percent of a pound?)

Baking recipes elsewhere generally use metric weight measures, too, for the same reason. Making these recipes consistent with recipes elsewhere means it's easier to compare them.

If you are interested in baking, or even just in cooking, and you don't have a digital scale, I would highly recommend that you get one. They are quite affordable these days, and once you have one, you will find more and more uses for it.

If you choose to use the Imperial measurements, you may need to do more adjusting to get these recipes to work well for you.

Health and Tradition

Nutrition is another reason to favor sourdough. Compared to "regular" bread, the longer ferment of sourdough does a better job of breaking down the phytic acid that occurs naturally in the flour, making it easier for our bodies to absorb nutrients. The longer ferment can also help break down the gluten proteins found in many grains. The longer the gluten proteins ferment, the more bioavailable they become, and the fewer problems they cause for people who are sensitive to them.

There is also a sense of a connection with history and with a tradition going back thousands of years. And there is the knowledge that in the event of infrastructure disruption, if it becomes difficult to get commercial yeast, we can continue to make bread. This was the situation at the beginning of the COVID-19 pandemic and part of what renewed my interest in sourdough.

Sourdough Starter

PREP TIME: 20–50 MINUTES, EPISODIC • TOTAL TIME: 4–10 DAYS

The sourdough starter is the basis for all sourdough recipes. You may already have a sourdough starter, you may be able to get some from a friend, or you could even buy some. But you can also produce your own, literally out of thin air. It's easy, and it's worth knowing how to do.

A sourdough starter is a living mixture of flour, water, yeast, and lactic and acetic acid-producing bacteria. It is somewhat analogous to a kombucha SCOBY (see page 100). The starter itself is most active at (warm) room temperature and at a somewhat goopy state of hydration, but it can survive in an impressive variety of environments and states.

Regardless of how you get your starter, the maintenance procedure ("feeding") is the same and is described below. Gradually you will get a better idea what sort of feeding works for your schedule, your temperament, and your starter. A lot of different routines can work—sourdough starters can be quite robust.

INGREDIENTS

At least 500 g (1 pound) flour, divided

Water (filtered, chlorine-free if possible)

EQUIPMENT

Quart or 1½-pint (1-L or ¾-L) mason jar with lid

Electronic scale

Canning funnel (optional)

—

Yield: Varies

PREPARATION

1. Remove the lid from the jar and put the jar on the scale, with the canning funnel if you are using one. Zero the scale.

2. "Feeding:" Add approximately 50 g (6½ tablespoons) of flour to the jar, then add an equal weight of water; stir them together vigorously using a clean spoon of some sort, or close the lid tightly and shake the jar if it seems like that will mix them well enough.

3. Leave the lid on the jar, tightly enough to keep critters out and to minimize evaporation but loosely enough to allow the contents to release gases if needed.

4. Every day, "feed" the jar more flour and water by following step 2 above.

5. After some number of days, the mixture will become bubbly and develop air pockets and a yeasty smell. It will be noticeable. At this point, you have succeeded in creating a sourdough starter! If you're not sure, then it hasn't happened yet. Keep going.

6. If the mixture hasn't gotten bubbly after several days and the jar is getting full, then dispose of most of the mixture, keeping an inch (2.5 cm) or so at the bottom, and continue feeding as before. Eventually it will start getting bubbly.

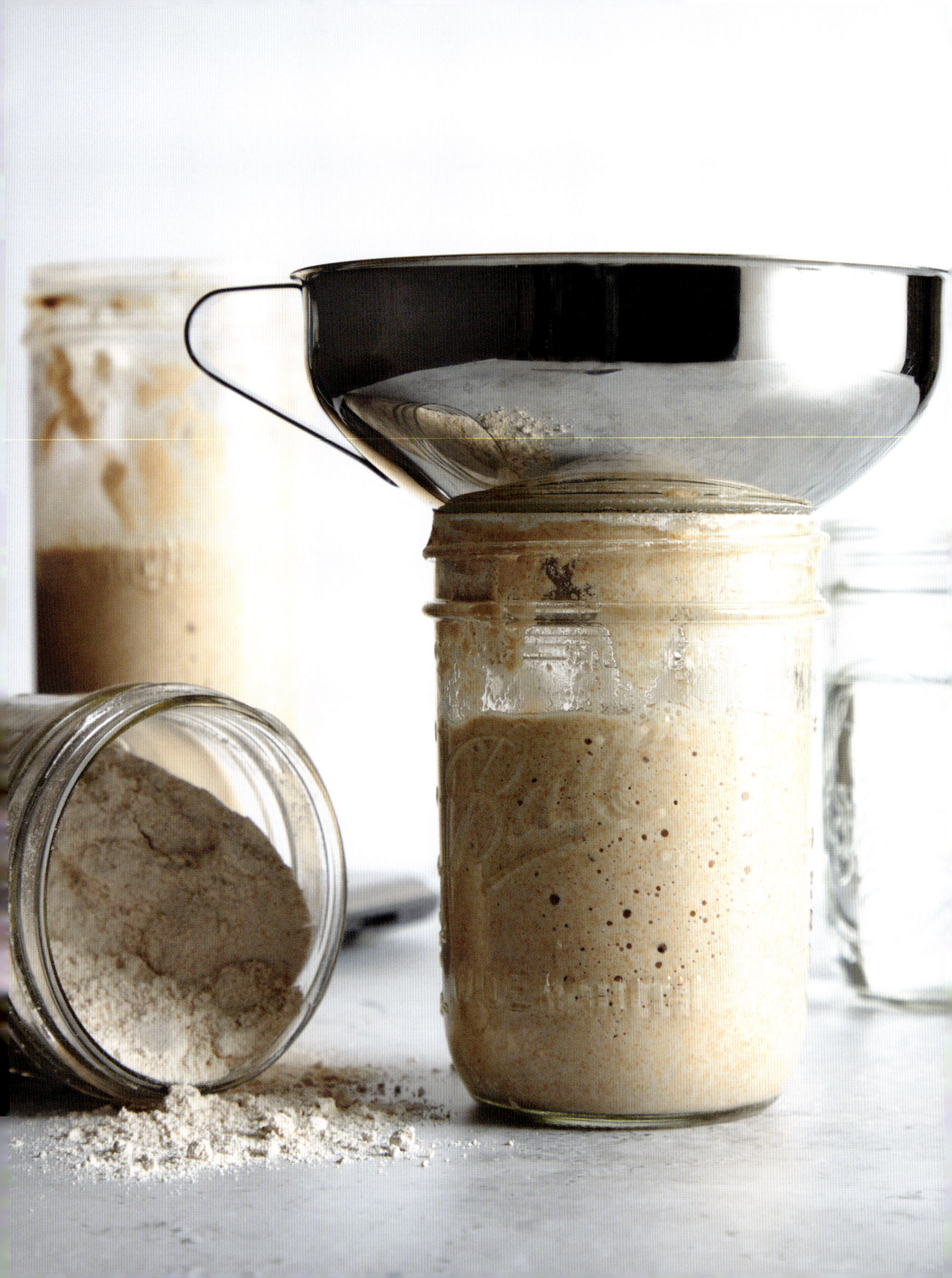

Care and Feeding

Once you have an established starter, you will need to feed it every day or two, depending on how frequently you use it and depending on other factors like ambient temperature (if the weather is hot, your starter may need to be fed every day).

To feed the starter, remove and set aside ("discard") half or more of the contents of the jar. You don't have to be precise about this. When I do it, I may tighten the lid, give it a good shake, open the lid, and then pour out the part that pours or as much as I want to pour out, leaving what's on the sides and on the bottom. Or maybe I'll give it a stir or a scrape around the sides with a knife.

Amount of Feeding

Once you have set aside your "discard," add equal amounts of flour and water by weight as in step 2 above. Ideally the amount you add will be equal to or greater than the amount already in the jar. For example, if you have less than or equal to 100 g (¾ cup) of starter left in the jar, then you can feed it with 50 g (6½ tablespoons) or more of flour and an equal weight of water. Then the next time you feed your starter, you can set aside the same amount that you added (100 g [¾ cup] or more) and feed similarly. One hundred grams (¾ cup) happens to be the amount of starter needed for the first two recipes below. If you want to bake bread, you will need about twice that, so you'll want to do a bigger feeding beforehand (generally eight hours or so before you start making the bread).

Discard with a Firm Hand

You may have an urge to "discard" as little as possible and keep as much of the nice bubbly sourdough bubbling as you can. Do not succumb to this urge! This is a mistake for two reasons: First of all, there are lots of delicious things you can do with the "discard"; you don't have to throw it away. (In fact, I have kept sourdoughs for long periods of time without making bread—simply making crackers, porridge, or other things with the discard.) Second, if you want a vigorous starter, less is more. It's better to feed a lot of flour and water to a little starter than to feed a little food to a lot of starter. A good guideline is that the feeding should be at least as big as the starter.

Rate of Feeding

As far as frequency goes, if feeding every day or two seems ambitious, you can also feed the sourdough and then put it in the refrigerator, where it will need to be fed only occasionally.

A NOTE ABOUT FLOUR

You can start a sourdough with one type of flour and feed it with a different one, or use a starter made with one flour to make a bread using mostly a different type of flour, etc. These days I find myself keeping a spelt sourdough starter and using it to bake bread with organic white (all-purpose) flour. You can experiment.

Especially if you are using white all-purpose flour, I would recommend buying organic flour or buying flour from a local mill. Less mainstream flours are premium products, may be grown with fewer herbicides and pesticides than their mainstream counterparts, and will make a nicer bread.

HYDRATION

You may see recipes elsewhere calling for "100% hydration sourdough starter." This means that the amount of water used is 100 percent of the amount of flour (they're equal). A "75% hydration starter," for instance, would have 75 g of water for every 100 g of flour.

The recipes here all use 100% hydration starter. In general, unless specified otherwise, sourdough recipes assume 100% hydration starter.

Take it out a couple of days before you'll need it for a project and then revive it with a couple of feedings. I'll only do this if I'm going to be out of town for an extended period. Otherwise, I just keep it on the counter. And if I'm going somewhere with a functioning kitchen, I might also take some starter, in a small container with my toiletries if I'm flying, and start feeding it at my destination. (I have not tried using sourdough starter as a facial mask, but others have, with good results. So if airport security questions your cosmetics, don't hesitate to rub your sourdough on your face. What's left on the sides of the jar should be sufficient to build it back up when you reach your destination.)

Oops! Troubleshooting

I have neglected a sourdough at (cool) room temperature for as long as a couple of months without feeding it and subsequently resuscitated it. I don't recommend neglecting a starter intentionally, but if you do think you might suddenly be pulled away, then it's good to get into the habit of keeping the lid and lip of your jar clean, both to prevent the jar from crusting itself shut (I've had that happen) and to minimize the chances of mold and such. A wipe with a moist paper towel should do the trick to keep the lip of the jar clean.

If a starter does sit for a while, liquid can collect on the top of it and it can start to smell funny. At this point, the starter might not respond to its feedings.

When trying to revive an unhappy sourdough starter, my technique is as follows:

1. Add a small amount—just a spoonful or two—of the unhappy starter to a clean jar.

2. Give it a regular feeding (50 g [6½ tablespoons] flour + 50 g [3½ tablespoons] water).

3. Proceed as usual.

If the starter doesn't get bubbly within a day or so after this, then you may have to start over.

Discard/Opportunity

In sourdough circles, the part you remove before feeding is often called "sourdough discard." I prefer to call it "sourdough opportunity."

Sourdough opportunity is a fully sour 24-hour fermented grain, optimally nutritious and digestible when cooked, ready to be used as a starting point for sourdough crackers (recipe page 137), sweet or savory sourdough pancakes or waffles, or (easiest of all) as sourdough porridge (recipe page 137). Or a facial mask!

If you need to feed your starter but you don't have time to use the extra, you can save it up in the fridge for a big batch of something on the weekend.

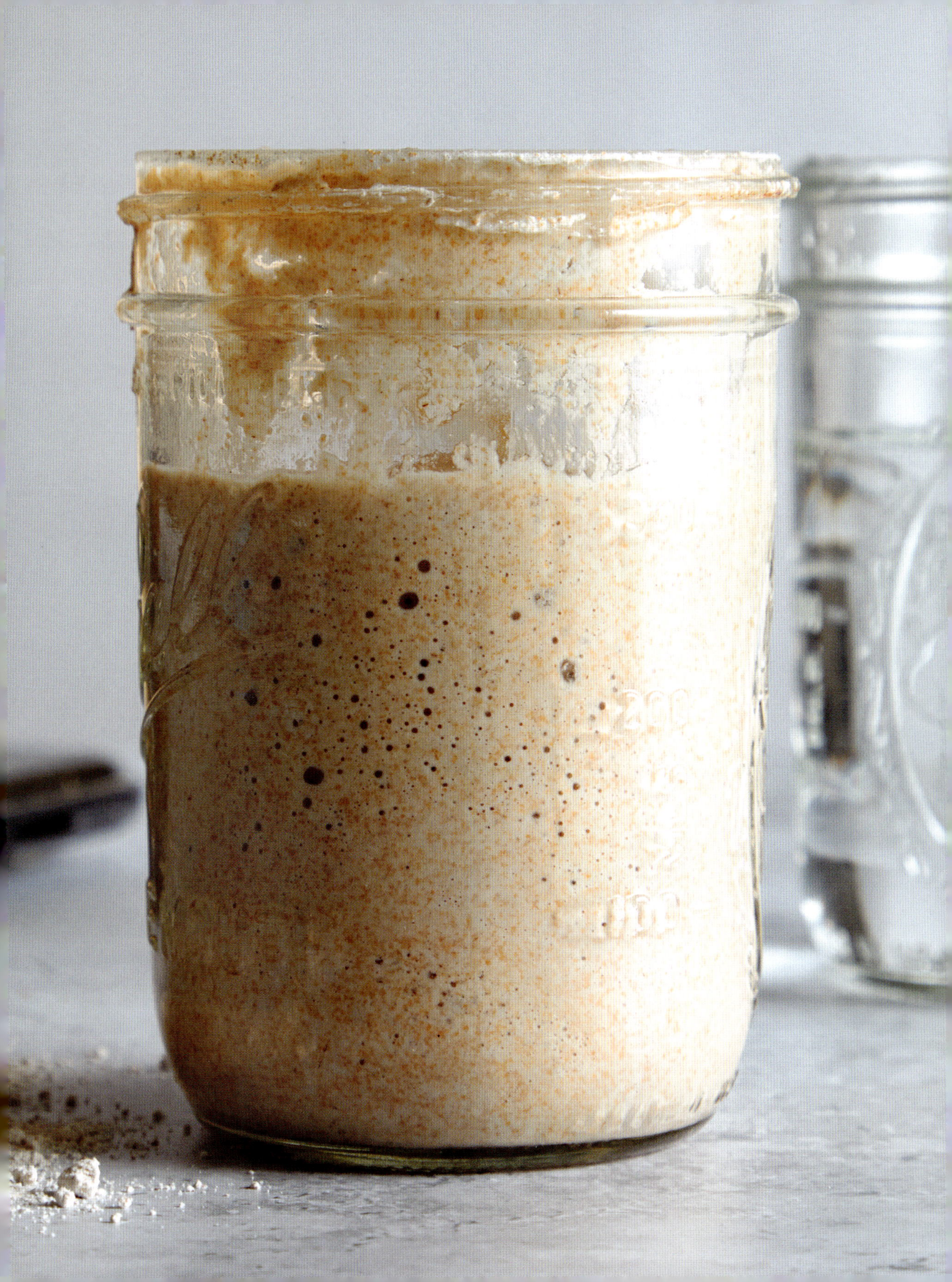

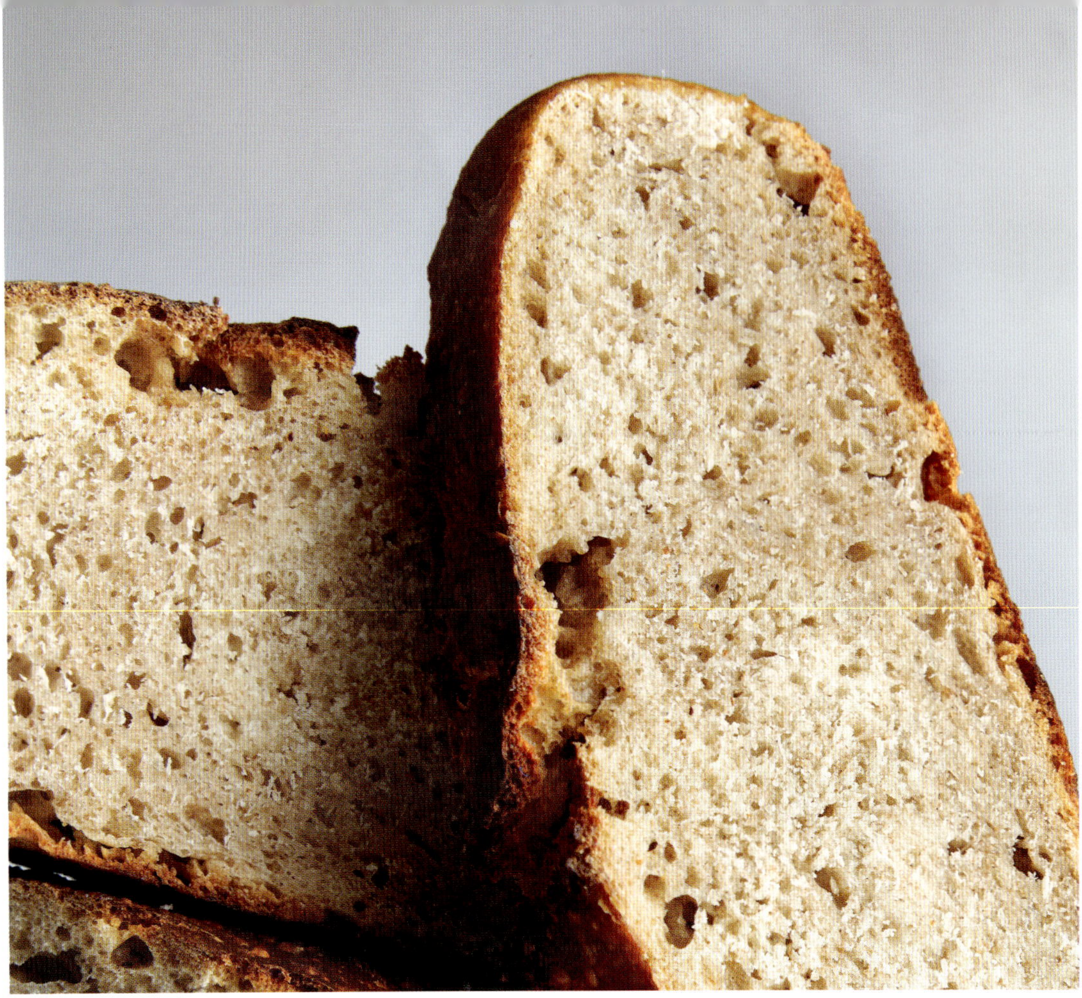

Sourdough Bread

PREP TIME: 30 MINUTES, EPISODIC • TOTAL TIME: AT LEAST 9 HOURS (VARIES)

This recipe reliably produces a medium-dense, chewy, flavorful loaf of bread for me. It's great as is or toasted. It's lovely on its own with some butter, or it can be used for a sandwich or *smørrebrød*. It also has a good shelf life.

The stand mixer in this recipe is not necessary, and purists might object—but it does make things easier and quicker.

Likewise, the Dutch oven is not necessary, but it helps make things more oven-independent and helps control temperature and humidity. The Dutch oven creates a humidity-controlled microclimate that is insulated from sudden temperature changes. Other options for managing humidity involve trays of water and spray bottles; I find these options less consistent and less convenient.

This recipe is just a starting point. If you like making sourdough bread, there are many more resources out there.

INGREDIENTS
225 g (¾ cup) starter (ideally fed approximately 8 hours before)

180 g (¾ cup) water

10 g (1½ teaspoons) salt

360 g (3 cups) white flour

1 teaspoon (4.5 ml) olive oil or other fat for greasing parchment

EQUIPMENT
5-quart (5-L) stand mixer with dough hook, or confidence making dough by hand

Small (approximately 3-quart [3-L]) (enameled or non-enameled) cast iron Dutch oven with a tight-fitting lid. (If you don't have a Dutch oven, you can use a stoneware casserole; it must be safe up to 500°F [260°C]. The stoneware won't hold temperature quite as well as the Dutch oven, but it will work fine.)

Two roundish pieces of parchment large enough to mostly line the bottom and sides of the Dutch oven

Small, clean, lightweight organic towel or shirt, moistened with water

Oven for baking (because of the Dutch oven, you may be able to get away with using a large, powerful toaster oven!)

A warm place for "proofing." This could be an oven with the oven light on or an oven with a "proof" setting if you have it, or perhaps a multicooker such as an Instant Pot with a "proof" or "yogurt" setting with adjustable temperature. Your target is 77°F (25°C). You can vary a bit in either direction.

continued

PREPARATION

1. Put starter, water, and salt in the bowl of a stand mixer. Mix until uniform. Add flour gradually or all at once and mix. You want it to form a ball of dough that mostly cleans the sides of the bowl. If it's too dry and crumbly, then add water, a little at a time, with the mixer going, until it comes together. If it's very wet, then add bits of flour. You may need to wrangle the dough a little to get it to stay in the bowl. This recipe may be on the large side for some smaller mixers. (If you have experience making dough by hand and you would like to, then do so, and skip the stand mixer!)

2. Turn off the mixer. Remove the bowl from the mixer. Handle the dough a bit. Push it into a rounded ball with your (clean) hands (a).

Put the parchment in the bottom of a metal bowl, grease it lightly to moderately, and put the dough on top of it (b). (This metal bowl can be your mixer bowl, if it will fit in your warm place. Otherwise, use a smaller metal bowl. But leave room for your dough to double in size.) If there is a lot of space between your dough and the top of the bowl, put a second piece of parchment loosely on top of the dough. Cover the top of the bowl with the moist towel.

3. Put the bowl with the covered dough in your warm place. Leave it there for about 8 hours. This is the "proofing" stage. Remove it from the warm place and have a look at the dough. It may or may not have doubled in size. Put it back where it was with the parchment and the towel.

continued

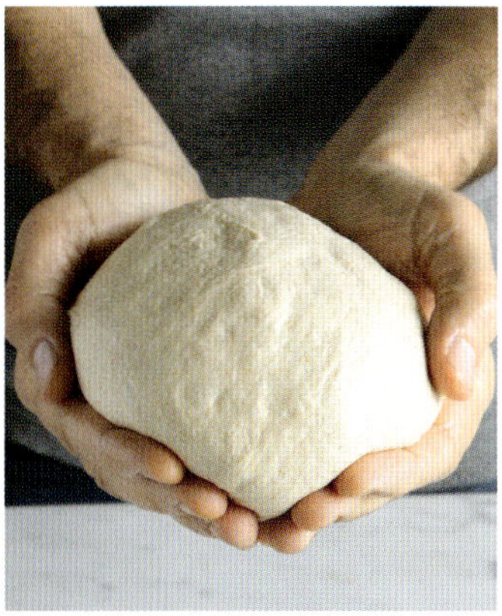

a

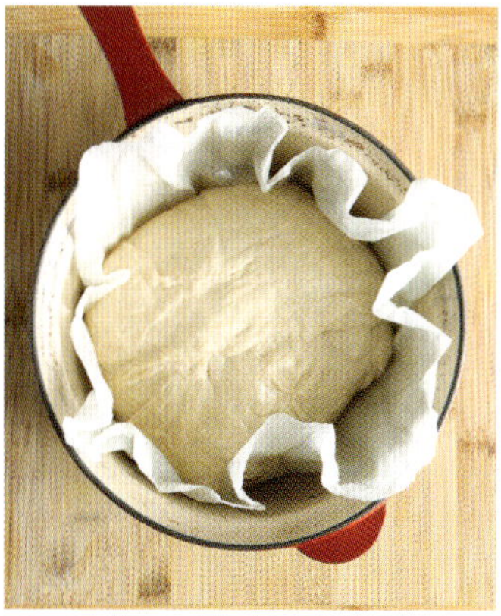

b

Sourdough Bread *(continued)*

A 2-quart (2-L) metal bowl for proofing (must be small enough to fit in your proofing place)

A cooling rack or equivalent (must allow air circulation underneath)

Heavy oven mitts or welding gloves

Instant-read food thermometer (recommended)

Oven thermometer (optional)

—

Yield: 1 medium-sized loaf

4. Put the Dutch oven and lid into the oven and heat the oven to 500°F (260°C). Once the oven is up to temperature, wait another 20 minutes to ensure that the Dutch oven is also up to temperature.

5. Find a heat-safe surface, like the top of a stove. With thick oven mitts, welding gloves, or the equivalent, remove the preheated Dutch oven and lid from the oven and put them on the heat-safe surface. Remove the moist towel and top parchment from the dough, lift the dough by the bottom parchment, and put it in the Dutch oven, with the parchment still underneath it. Watch it carefully—it will grow! Score the dough on top with a sharp knife or a pair of scissors if you like (see below).

Put the lid on the Dutch oven, put it back in the oven, and turn the oven temperature down to 450°F (230°C).

6. After 20 minutes, remove the Dutch oven from the oven, open the lid, and pull the bread out carefully. Remove the parchment now so that it doesn't stick to the bread or burn. Put the bread back in the Dutch oven with the lid off and put everything back in the oven for another 20 minutes.

7. Remove from oven.

If you have an instant-read thermometer, then take a temperature reading a third of the way down into the center of the loaf. If it's at 205°F (96°C) or above, remove it from the oven and take it out to

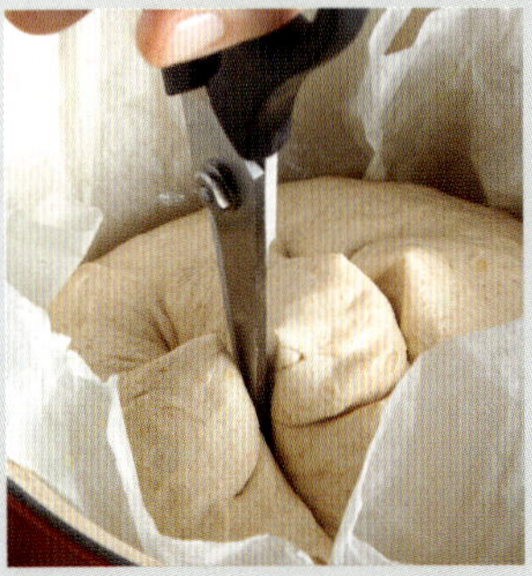

HERE'S THE EXPLANATION OF SCORING

The bread crust will crack open, somewhere, to let steam escape. If you score the bread, then you can guide this cracking; otherwise, the bread cracks open where it wants. If the sides of the bread were unsupported, it could crack open on the sides, which would not be ideal. But in our case, because of the Dutch oven, it will only crack open on the top anyway. So scoring is not necessary.

cool on the cooling rack. Otherwise, put it back in the oven with the lid off for another 10 minutes, then remove it and check the temperature again. Repeat until the bread reaches 205°F (96°C).

If you don't have an instant-read thermometer, then you can tap the bread on its underside; if it's done, it will make a hollow sound. This can work well if you are an experienced bread maker, but I still prefer using a thermometer—and using a thermometer makes the temperature check easier because you can leave the bread in the pot.

8. Let the bread cool on a cooling rack for 10 or 15 minutes or until it is close to room temperature.

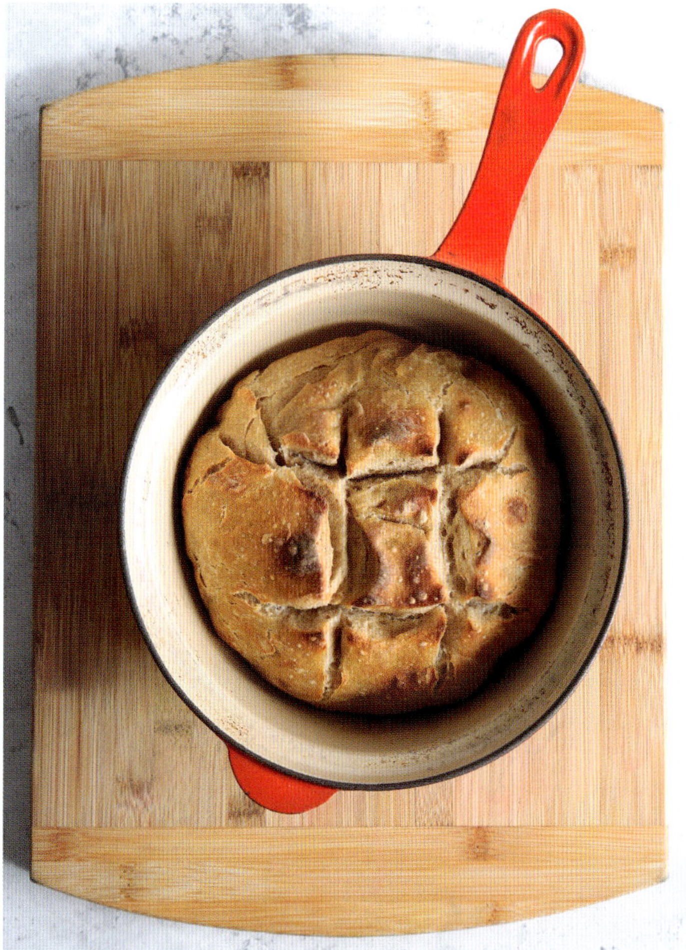

Sourdough Porridge

PREP TIME: 2 MINUTES • TOTAL TIME: 10 MINUTES

Porridges, sweet and savory, are staple foods around the world. They're eaten at various times of the day and go by too many names to list (porridge, poi, polenta, fufu, congee, etc.). Fermented porridges are common and get the nod for their superior nutrition and digestibility, and for their interesting sour flavor notes.

This recipe is an easy delicious use for sourdough discard. It has a nice sour flavor, and if made with spelt or other whole-grain discard, it has a nice depth to it. Depending how much liquid you add, it can be as thick or as thin as you like. A pinch of salt brings out the flavor.

It can be a vehicle for other ingredients you'd like to add, including fats, dairy, and sweeteners. I find myself making it most often with butter and molasses and sometimes a bit of dried fruit.

It's important that you keep your eye on it and stir it well as it's heating up. Failure to do so can result in lumpy porridge!

INGREDIENTS

100 g (or ⅓ cup) sourdough discard

240 g (or 1 cup) water

Pinch salt

Butter, coconut oil, ghee, or other delicious fat (optional)

Mineral-rich sweetener of choice, like molasses, honey, or maple syrup (optional)

Raisins or other dried or fresh fruit (optional)

Milk, cream, yogurt, crème fraîche, or other dairy (optional)

Replace some of the water with beer (try something dark; avoid anything very bitter), or with bread kvass or Malta (optional, "Øllebrød-style")

EQUIPMENT

Small/medium saucepan

Spoon or silicone spatula

—

Yield: One serving

PREPARATION

1. Add water and discard to pan. Stir.

2. Heat over medium heat, stirring frequently to quell lumps.

3. Once it's bubbling uniformly, reduce heat but keep it bubbling to ensure it cooks for five or more minutes. Cover if desired.

4. Remove from heat and add salt and optional ingredients.

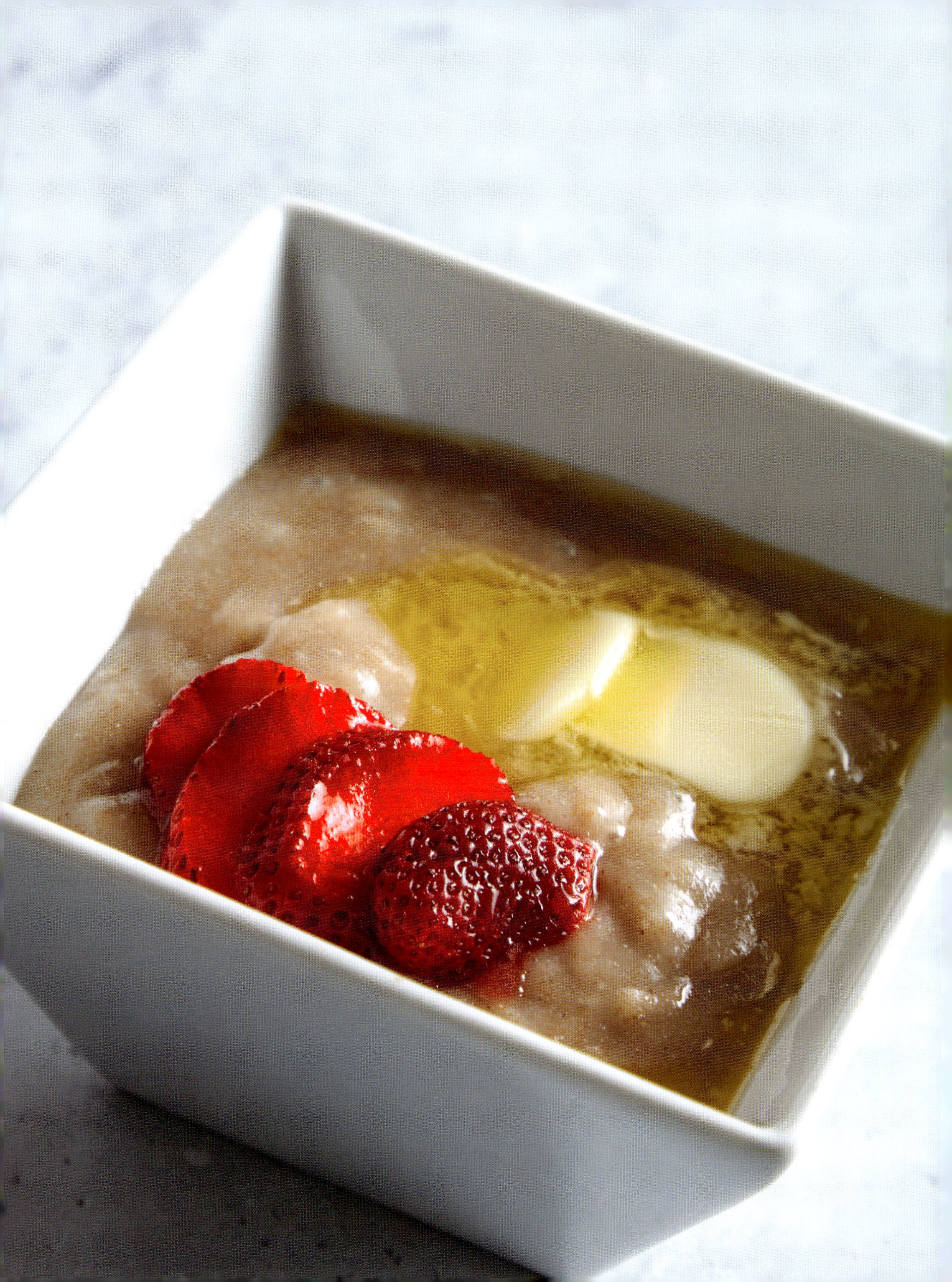

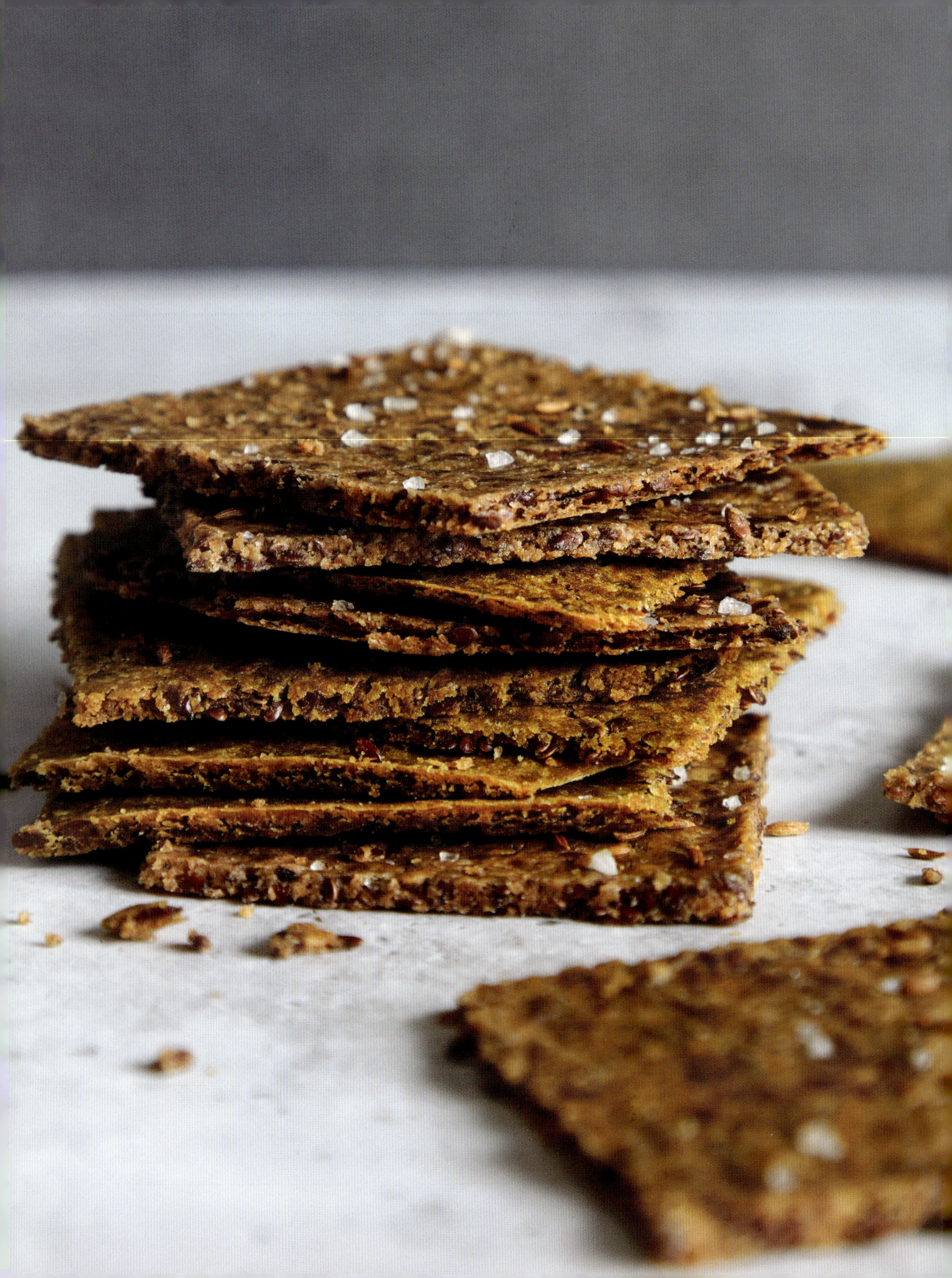

Sourdough Flax Crackers

PREP TIME: 7 MINUTES TOTAL TIME: APPROXIMATELY 90 MINUTES (VARIES)

I was making these crackers every day for a while. They are tasty enough that they can be eaten on their own as snacks. Cumin and curry powder have been my go-to flavors—use what you like and what you have, and do not be shy with the seasoning, including the salt.

When done, the crackers will be gratifyingly crispy without being at all burnt. The low temperature given in the recipe is necessary to avoid burning the crackers, especially if you are including the flaxseeds.

This was inspired in part by Sandor Katz's Flax Crackers recipe.

INGREDIENTS

100 g sourdough discard

100 g (about ¾ cup) soaked whole flaxseeds (see below)

25 g (two scant tablespoons) olive oil

Water as needed

Fennel seeds, cumin seeds or ground cumin, curry powder, Italian seasoning, Herbes de Provence, and/or other spices and herbs. A tablespoon of herbs or a teaspoon of spices is a good starting point. Adjust as you like in subsequent batches.

Some fancy salt and/or additional seeds as toppers (optional)

EQUIPMENT

Smallish mixing bowl

Silicone spatula

Quarter-sheet baking pan (9.5" × 13" [24 × 33 cm]) lined with a silicone baking mat or parchment

Oven (or toaster oven)

—

Yield: 12 3" × 3" (7.5 × 7.5 cm) crackers

PREPARATION

PREPARATION OF SOAKED FLAXSEEDS

In a pint jar, mix ½ cup (75 g) whole flaxseeds with ½ cup (120 ml) of salty water-based liquid. This is a great use for leftover pickle or sauerkraut brine; plain brine is a possibility, too (1 teaspoon [6 g] salt). Cover and refrigerate for at least a couple of hours until mucilaginous, or for up to a week.

PREPARATION OF SOURDOUGH FLAX CRACKERS

1. Add all ingredients to the mixing bowl except the toppers. Mix well. Add little bits of water as needed until the mixture is pourable but not watery.

2. Pour the mixture onto the lined baking pan. Spread to uniform thickness with spatula if needed. (If it is too difficult to get it to uniform thickness, then put it back in the mixing bowl, add more water, and try this step again.)

3. Bake at 250°F (120°C) (with convection if you have it) for 10 minutes. There's no need to preheat. Remove the pan from the oven and place it on a heat-safe surface.

4. Using the edge of the spatula or the blunt side of a knife, score the crackers-in-progress in both directions to achieve the desired individual cracker size. Two scores the long way and three the short way yields 12 approximately 3" × 3" (7.5 × 7.5 cm) crackers.

Sourdough Flax Crackers *(continued)*

LAB NOTES

If you don't want to use flaxseeds, you can make this recipe with all sourdough, with the following changes:

(1) 200 g (⅔ cup) sourdough instead of 100 g (⅓ cup) starter + 100 g (¾ cup) flax;

(2) add 1 teaspoon (6 g) of salt along with the spices; and

(3) oven can be 275°F (135°C) instead of 250°F (120°C).

5. At this point, sprinkle the optional extra salt and/or seeds across the top as uniformly as possible and seat them gently with your fingertips.

6. Return the crackers to the oven and continue baking at 250°F (120°C) for 20-minute intervals, checking the crackers each time, turning the pan 180° each time, and repeating until the crackers are dry and crispy. Loosen the crackers from the pan liner at the first moment when they seem willing to come off cleanly, then let them continue to bake. Break them along the score lines when you can to help the landlocked crackers cook more quickly.

7. When done, remove crackers from liner and pan. Let cool. Break along score lines if you haven't already. Store in an airtight container.

IS SOURDOUGH A FAD?

Today, it may be tempting to call sourdough bread a "fad" because, like kombucha, kimchi, and the others, it has become the subject of much attention. It may also be tempting to call sourdough bread "elite" and to view it as some sort of class marker, since sourdough bread is more expensive to buy than "regular" bread and more difficult and time-consuming to make.

The truth is that for most of the history of bread, *all* leavened bread was "sourdough." Packaged yeast did not exist until the late nineteenth century!

Sourdough bread has been perfectly mainstream at particular times in particular places. The change we're seeing now is that we are becoming increasingly aware of what exactly we're eating and how it was made.

Resources

Some of the resources below are mentioned in this book. This resource list can also be found online at http://RealFoodFermentation.com/resources, where all the items are clickable. The online version of this list will be updated regularly and will continue to grow.

BOOKS

Appetite for Change: How the Counterculture Took on the Food Industry by Warren Belasco. A fascinating documentation of the ongoing culture war surrounding access to food.

Home Cheese Making by Ricki Carroll. The reference how-to book by the person who started the modern small-scale cheese-making movement in the United States.

The Jungle: The Uncensored Original Edition by Upton Sinclair. A singular document of the horrors of the early industrial meat industry, unexpurgated and as the author intended it to be read.

The Kimchi Chronicles: Korean Cooking for an American Kitchen by Maria Vongerichten. A beautiful book that includes a lot of ideas for how to cook with one of our favorite fermented foods.

Kombucha: Healthy Beverage and Natural Remedy from the Far East by Günter Frank. A meticulous and thorough book about the "dos" and "don'ts" of making kombucha.

The Long Emergency: Surviving the End of Oil, Climate Change, and Other Converging Catastrophes of the Twenty-First Century by James Howard Kunstler. A convincing case for the urgency of the problems facing our world, and why you should learn to make your own food!

Manifestos on the Future of Food and Seed edited by Vandana Shiva. A collection of compelling essays on the problems of modern industrial food, and a bold attempt to solve these problems.

Meat: A Benign Extravagance by Simon Fairlie. The author makes a meticulously crafted argument that meat production and consumption can be environmentally sound, even advantageous, if done properly.

Milk: The Surprising Story of Milk Through the Ages by Anne Mendelson. Everything you never knew you didn't know about milk and dairy, including recipes, in a thoroughly entertaining and lovely book.

Nourishing Traditions: The Cookbook that Challenges Politically Correct Nutrition and the Diet Dictocrats by Sally Fallon Morell and Mary G. Enig. The best modern nutrition writing I've come across—followed by a unique description of a wide range of traditional food preparations.

Nutrition and Physical Degeneration by Weston A. Price. Dr. Price's detective work uncovers 14 isolated groups of people with exemplary health, and finds and documents commonalities among their diets.

On Food and Cooking: The Science and Lore of the Kitchen by Harold McGee. The modern food science reference. Anyone wanting to know about the "why" of food can get this book, and chances are they will find their answers within.

The Raw Milk Revolution by David Gumpert. A very engaging window on the current ongoing battles between food regulators and big business on one side and individuals and small farmers on the other over the question of who gets to decide what foods are legal and illegal, written with the pace of a good thriller.

The Revolution Will Not Be Microwaved: Inside America's Underground Food Movements by Sandor Katz. Reading this book helped me understand how all the pieces of the food puzzle fit together, and along the way managed to excite and move me more than any book in recent memory—informative, authentic, and passionate.

Seeds of Deception: Exposing Industry and Government Lies About the Safety of the Genetically Engineered Foods You're Eating by Jeffrey M. Smith. A provocative look at the increasing evidence that genetically modified foods are a growing disaster.

ServSafe Coursebook by Association Solutions National Restaurant Association. This is the United States food industry reference on food safety.

Silent Spring by Rachel Carson. The book that started the modern environmental movement.

Wild Fermentation: The Flavor, Nutrition, and Craft of Live-Culture Foods by Sandor Katz. An awesome look at the ancient art of fermentation and its place in the context of our modern existence, including lots of recipes. A must-have for any serious—or even casual—fermenter. The book that put sauerkraut back on the map.

FILMS

Farmageddon (2011). Kristin Canty sheds light on egregious over reaches by regulatory and law enforcement agencies, creating and imposing unreasonable policies at the expense of farmers and private individuals.

Food, Inc. (2008). Exposes how modern food production feeds the wallets of food industry hegemons at the expense of ordinary, particularly rural, and lower-income people.

Fresh (2009). Exposes some of the problems with our food system, and highlights some of the innovative solutions that people are coming up with.

The Future of Food (2004). Director Deborah Koons Garcia presents a disturbing picture of food technology trends and their impact on society and the environment.

The World According to Monsanto (2008). Filmmaker Marie-Monique Robin tells a disturbing story of collusion between industry and government to control food production at its very root: the farm.

ORGANIZATIONS

Cornucopia Institute. Seeking economic justice for the family-scale farming community. They provide a plethora of useful information about food—for instance, an egg-buying guide that goes beyond "free-range," "cage-free," and "organic."

Environmental Working Group. A group focused on environmental toxins. Their "Clean 15/Dirty Dozen" shopper's guide is a great outline of which foods are most important to buy organic.

Weston A. Price Foundation. A fantastic, fast-growing non-profit foundation dedicated to restoring healthy, nutrient-dense, real food to the human diet. Their website is a treasure trove of information about food, diet, and physiology.

OTHER BLOGS AND WEBSITES

The Complete Patient. David Gumpert's blog defines the cutting edge of raw milk and food freedom journalism.

Feed Me Like You Mean It. My blog where I talk about fermentation, real food, raw milk, and where it's all leading, with some recipes.

Kombucha Fuel. Annabelle Ho's blog follows her extensive experience brewing kombucha, doing live demonstrations, and documenting other kombucha-related events.

Real Food Media. A network of first-rate bloggers who provide inspiring and informative recipes, stories, and commentary on the subject of real food.

FOOD PRODUCERS, STORES, AND SCHOOLS

The Cheese School of San Francisco. A great cheese-making school in the heart of San Francisco, California

Filters Fast. This is where I have bought my water filtration systems.

Giant Microbes. Stuffed animals, but instead of animals they're microbes. Buy one to make sure you don't raise bacteriophobes.

The Homebrew Emporium. A great place for brewing-related gear.

New England Cheesemaking Supply Company. Ricki Carroll's unique cheese-making school, and an online resource for cheese-making supplies.

Taza Chocolate. A cutting-edge, small batch chocolate producer.

About the Author

Alex Lewin has always loved food, eating, experiments, and puzzles.

After studying math at Harvard and working in the computer industry, he became more and more interested in food and health, in particular the question of what to eat. Buy ten books about diet, and they will tell you ten different things. Why is this?

Cooking school (Cambridge School of Culinary Arts) and nutrition school (Institute for Integrative Nutrition) helped Alex frame general answers: Some of the things that we eat today are simply toxic; different people need different kinds of foods; and, sadly, much of the food and health industry is driven by money and ambition rather than science, wisdom, or compassion.

In order to create a healthier and tastier world, Alex spreads the good news about fermentation, by writing about it here and in his blog, and by teaching fermentation classes and leading workshops. He also serves on the board of the Boston Public Market Association, working to create a year-round indoor market selling local food.

At his day job, Alex writes software, averts disasters, and generally tries to create order out of chaos.

Besides food, health, and computers, his interests include music, all manner of two-wheeled vehicles, cats, and exploring the obscure. He lives in Oakland and Cambridge.

To find out more, visit his blog at http://RealFoodFermentation.com.

Index

T

U

V

W

Y